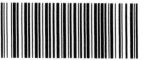

If Memory Serves

IF MEMORY SERVES

Gay Men, AIDS, and the Promise
of the Queer Past

CHRISTOPHER CASTIGLIA *and*
CHRISTOPHER REED

University of Minnesota Press
Minneapolis
London

An earlier version of chapter 1 was published as Christopher Castiglia, "Sex Publics, Sex Panics, Sex Memories," *boundary 2* 27, no. 2 (Summer 2000): 149–75; and as Christopher Castiglia, "The Way We Were: Remembering the Gay 70s," in *The Seventies: The Age of Glitter in Popular Culture*, ed. Shelton Waldrep (New York: Routledge, 1999), 206–23. An earlier version of chapter 2 was published as Christopher Reed, "Imminent Domain: Queer Space in the Built Environment," *Art Journal* 55, no. 4 (Winter 1996): 64–70; Christopher Reed, "We're from Oz: Marking Ethnic and Sexual Identity," *Environment and Planning D: Society and Space* 21, no. 4 (August 2003): 425–40; and Christopher Reed, "A Third Chicago School?" in *Chicago Architecture: Histories, Revisions, Alternatives*, ed. Katerina Rae Reudi and Charles Waldheim (Chicago: University of Chicago Press, 2005), 163–75. An earlier version of chapter 3 was published as Christopher Castiglia and Christopher Reed, "'Ah Yes, I Remember It Well': Memory, Mass Media, and *Will and Grace*," *Cultural Critique* 56 (Winter 2004): 158–88. An earlier version of chapter 4 was published as Christopher Castiglia, "Past Burning: The (Post)Traumatic Crisis of (Post-) Queer Theory," in *States of Emergency*, ed. Russ Castronovo and Susan Gillman (Chapel Hill: University of North Carolina Press, 2009), 69–87.

Published by the University of Minnesota Press
111 Third Avenue South, Suite 290
Minneapolis, MN 55401-2520
http://www.upress.umn.edu

Library of Congress Cataloging-in-Publication Data

Castiglia, Christopher.
    If memory serves : gay men, AIDS, and the promise of the queer past /
Christopher Castiglia and Christopher Reed.
        p.   cm.
    Includes bibliographical references and index.
    ISBN 978-0-8166-7610-1 (hc : alk. paper)
    ISBN 978-0-8166-7611-8 (pb : alk. paper)
    1. Gays — United States — History.   2. Gay culture — United States — History.
3. AIDS (Disease) — Social aspects — United States.   4. Queer theory — United States.
5. Gay and lesbian studies — United States.   I. Reed, Christopher, 1961–   II. Title.
    HQ76.3.U5.C375   2012
    306.76'60973 — dc23
                                                                                2011031750

Printed in the United States of America on acid-free paper

The University of Minnesota is an equal-opportunity educator and employer.

18 17 16 15 14 13 12   10 9 8 7 6 5 4 3 2

Dedicated to the memory of our teachers and friends,
John Boswell and Vito Russo,
and to Simon Watney,
who continues to teach and inspire us.

CONTENTS

INTRODUCTION

In the Interest of Time

Memory is the diary that chronicles things that never happened
or couldn't possibly have happened.

—OSCAR WILDE

Unremembering

About the time we started talking about the ideas in this book, we were
getting ready to move for a year to Memphis, Tennessee. Looking up gay
life there, we found the most popular gay club in Memphis was called
Amnesia. Despite being heralded as "the Club for the new Millennium,"
by the time we arrived in Memphis, Amnesia had closed.[1] Something about
the vast, empty building and the even vaster empty parking lot—gay space
in the process of reverting to generic mid-American sprawl—seemed
disturbingly apt. It's hard to resist the allegory: offering flashy promise of
a guaranteed future (a club for the next millennium), A/amnesia produced
instead assimilation and loss in the place where a gay cultural life once
thrived. It's uncertain, of course, whether a nightclub named Recollection
or a piano bar called Memories would have fared any better. What is certain, we argue in the following chapters, is that the sacrifice of spaces and
rituals of memory to the lure of amnesia has weakened gay communities,
both our connections to one another and our ability to imagine, collectively and creatively, alternative social presents and futures for ourselves.

1

"The possession of an historical identity and the possession of a social identity coincide." This passage from the philosopher Alasdair MacIntyre's theorization of virtue has been influentially deployed by Gary Younge in relation to racial identity.[2] MacIntyre's point that "the self has to find its moral identity in and through membership in communities" is equally applicable to the sexual subject positions described by terms like "gay" and "queer," although the competition between those terms is itself an indication of the impetus toward forgetting that characterizes our recent history.[3] This problem is not ours alone. Gore Vidal coined the phrase "the United States of Amnesia" to evoke a national propensity to forget episodes that do not accord with our self-image (*Point to Point Navigation*, 55), and historian Tony Judt has characterized the era from the fall of the Berlin Wall in 1989 to the invasion of Iraq as a time when "we have become stridently insistent — in our economic calculations, our political practices, our international strategies, even our educational priorities — that *the past has nothing of interest to teach us*" (*Reappraisals*, 2). In this context, "forgetting" has attracted its own theoretical champions, who argue, in Andreas Huyssen's words, against "an omnipresent, even excessive public memory discourse and its mass marketing" ("Resistance to Memory," 182). These analyses make clear how today even the language of memory becomes a force for amnesia as certain "right" memories, in Huyssen's words, "are codified into national consensus and become clichés" (182).[4] This deployment of officially sanctioned narratives that picture the past to justify the norms of the present was analyzed by Foucault, who described how in France such sanctioned memories of World War II "obstruct the flow" of "popular memory" ("Film and Popular Memory," 91). Paradoxically, then, official memories — in the form of films, education, museum exhibitions, holidays, news reporting, and political speeches — constitute a potent form of forgetting even as they purport to traffic in memory. The assault on gay memory following AIDS took precisely this form, offering "cleaned-up" versions of the past as substitutes for more challenging memories of social struggle. What separates unremembering from such national amnesia, however, is the direct assault on particular memories and on the cultural act of remembering. Such attacks sought not to cohere an imagined national community but to undo the historical basis for communities that once seemed to offer radically new forms of social and sexual engagement.

Gay culture has been prey to a particularly intense version of un-remembering since the onset in the early 1980s of the AIDS epidemic. We are not saying that AIDS itself did in gay culture, although the very real costs of the syndrome in both human and financial terms has been staggering. Rather, the AIDS crisis became an occasion for a powerful concentration of cultural forces that made (and continue to make) the syndrome an agent of amnesia, wiping out memories not only of every-thing that came before but of the remarkably vibrant and imaginative ways that gay communities responded to the catastrophe of illness and death and sought to memorialize our losses.

As we show in chapter 1, "Battles over the Gay Past: De-generation and the Queerness of Memory," gay neocons in the 1990s promised that by making a complete break with a "diseased" past of narcissistic and reck-lessly immature pleasures that supposedly led to AIDS, gay men could achieve a maturity cast as normalcy that would safeguard health and pur-chase, sometime in the unspecified future, a place at the table of politi-cal negotiations. Echoing the newly politicized Christian fundamentalist preachers who were achieving unprecedented prominence at the same period, gay neoconservatives recast sexual revolution as a dangerous form of immaturity.[5] The sexual past was relentlessly reconfigured as a site of infectious irresponsibility rather than valued for generating and main-taining the systems of cultural communication and care that proved the best — often the only — response to disease, backlash, and death. Advo-cates of amnesia, prescribing normalcy in the benevolent-sounding lan-guage of public safety, rationalized the regulation and closure of spaces of gay sexual culture.[6] But as the far-reaching, socially transformative de-mands associated with early gay liberation and AIDS activism shrank to agendas organized around conformity to institutionalized authority vested in church, state, and science — campaigns to win the right to marry, to join the military, or to "cure" gender dysphoria — we began to wonder what model of "health" amnesia, in the end, procures.

Of course, the neocon agenda was contested, as we also show through-out the book. Even as activists and academics challenged the pathologized depictions of the sexual past, however, the 1990s saw the rise of less ob-viously prescriptive forms of forgetting, demonstrating what Roderick Ferguson describes as "the ways in which normativity attempts to close off prior critical and sexual universes" by transforming past struggles "into historic quests for legitimacy and evaluating legitimacy through how well we surrender claims to sex and sexual heterogeneity" ("Theorizing Queer Temporalities," 193). Vincent Doyle documents one exemplary instance of unremembering within GLAAD (Gay and Lesbian Alliance Against Defamation), the political organization charged, ironically, with protecting gays and lesbians from discriminatory misrepresentation. Throughout the 1990s, GLAAD underwent a process of professionalization, replacing founding members who came from the ranks of the 1970s Gay Activist Alliance with media executives and lawyers. That transformation, Doyle argues, was accompanied by a self-justifying refiguring of the organization's past as having been always dedicated to "visibility politics." This reconfiguration of the past, Doyle contends, was "a kind of structurally embedded amnesia, a strategic forgetting" that took GLAAD "away from the confrontation with dominant institutions toward the supposed equality that visibility politics continually promises but perpetually defers" ("'But Joan!'" 210). Enabled by "historical amnesia," Doyle reports, what struck GLAAD's founding members as a hostile takeover "felt to the movement's new entrants like a historically sanctioned handover" (213). For Doyle, the stakes of such amnesia extend beyond questions of historical accuracy to engage "nothing less than the future of our capacity to imagine new political and cultural possibilities beyond the limits of mainstreaming" (220).

Similar forms of professionalization marked the transformation of early gay and lesbian studies into the first wave of "queer theory" in the academy. Although second-wave work in queer theory—historically grounded, socially engaged, multiethnic, and sensitive to the spatial and temporal operations of sexuality—has helped us formulate our investigation of coercive unremembering and queer countermemory here, earlier instantiations of queerness, in the academy and outside it, made claims to radicalism that often comprised nothing more radical than their disavowal of caricatures of an older generation's supposedly monolithic and naively "essentialist" constructions of sexual identity. Elizabeth Freeman rightly observes that in academia, "whatever looks newer or more-radical-than-thou has more purchase over prior signs, and that whatever seems to generate continuity seems better left behind" ("Packing History, Count(er)ing Generations," 728). This strategy of chronological one-upmanship is hardly unique to the theorization of sexuality; the institutionalization of "theory" in general often manifests the way "the academic psyche has internalized the fashion system," as Bill Brown pithily puts it ("Thing Theory," 13). But as we show in chapter 4, "Queer Theory Is Burning: Sexual Revolution and Traumatic Unremembering," well-received versions of queer theory in the 1990s often signaled their novelty in ways that participated in post-AIDS unremembering and, at the same time, registered the traumatic aftereffects of their own unremembering. Our skepticism focuses on how minority sexual cultures were academically institutionalized at the cost of our own histories, as early versions of queer theory, replacing an oversimplified notion of "identity" with a dehistoricized psyche or with decollectivizing, shame-inducing, or ego-shattering death drives, made a point of unremembering the joyous, collective, idealistic, and socially situated possibilities of sexual liberation and the integration of activism and scholarship that characterized practices formulated under the rubric of "gay" and "lesbian." To be clear, our complaint is not a generational one about the disrespect young scholars show older ones. On the contrary, we relish the skepticism toward some of the axioms of liberationist politics and participate in many of the intellectual endeavors classed under "queer theory." What we *are* contending is that the first wave of queer theory, like any discursive formation, arose at a particular moment for reasons other than greater intellectual acuity and that at least one of those reasons was the general unremembering that took hold in the aftershock of the first years of AIDS. It was that context that not only demanded a "queer subject," solitary and outside history, but that also detached itself from its intellectual roots in ways that made "gay theory" seem an anachronistic oxymoron.

The gesture of disavowing a gay past in order to procure a queer rigor carries through into projects with which we are otherwise sympathetic. José Esteban Muñoz's *Cruising Utopia: The Then and There of Queer Futurity*, for example, opens by defining "queerness" as "a doing for and toward the future"; thus, "we have never been queer" (1). Although Muñoz grounds his emphasis on "hope" in Ernst Bloch's theorization of how "hope's methodology (with its pendant, memory) dwells in the region of the not-yet" (3) and starts by locating "a modality of queer utopianism that I locate within a historically specific nexus of cultural production before, around, and slightly after the Stonewall rebellion of 1969," his engagement with the past is defensive and ambivalent. Muñoz casts his project as an "attempt to counteract the logic of the historical case study" with a rhetoric anxious to assert agency over a past he "tracks," "leaps" to, and "brings in" (3) — this in contrast to the queerness that "is not yet here but it approaches like a crashing wave of potentiality. And we must give in to its propulsion" (185).[7] In contrast to this utopian vision, the "kind of futurity" Muñoz finds in the pre-Stonewall past is deduced from its failures, as in the "semidisowned ending" of LeRoi Jones's (later Amiri Baraka) 1964 play *The Toilet,* in which a high-school boy cradles the battered head of a lover he has just helped to brutally fag-bash: this "moment of wounded recognition . . . tells us that this moment in time . . . is not all there is, that indeed something is missing," thus offering "a utopian kernel and an anticipatory illumination" (90–91). In this model, the past is valued mainly because it requires redemption by the future. Even more problematically, Muñoz asserts his bid for "queer utopia" in a way that unremembers the utopian aspects of gay (and lesbian) culture. Asserting "we were queer before we were lesbian or gay" (127), Muñoz asks readers to "reflect on what was lost" by the "turn to the identitarian" he associates with the "formalizing and formatting of gay and lesbian identities" he says took place soon after June of 1969 (115). Such rhetorical disavowals of the recent past set up Muñoz's interest in connecting a pre-Stonewall queer past with current manifestations of queerness in the New York and Los Angeles avant-gardes, undercutting the implications of his brief but eloquent analysis of a "radical and poignant" (197) manifesto, "What We Want, What We Believe," from the gay liberation journal *Gay Flames.* Drawing attention to the "we" of the "Third World Gay Revolution" collective that authored this manifesto, Muñoz revels in its articulation of demands "many people would dismiss . . . as impractical or utopian" consolidated by a "we" that "is not content to describe who the collective is but more nearly describes what the collective and the larger social order could be, what it should be" (19). Retrieving this articulation of "futurity" from the otherwise ignored 1970s, Muñoz is right to assert, "There is great value in pulling these words from the no-longer conscious to arm a critique of the present" (19), but is wrong in assuming that such traces of the past take on significance *only* when translated into present terms, that the *pastness* of memory does no important work of its own.

Muñoz's insistence that the "we" of this manifesto "does not speak to a merely identitarian logic" he associates with "identity politics" itself participates in an unremembering of the historical reliance *on* identity of such future-oriented radicalism. For Muñoz, groups like the Gay Liberation Front, which we further discuss in chapter 4, become radical only when taken from the context that gave rise to them (the identitarian movement Muñoz disavows) and translated into a present characterized by academic theory (supposedly, although very rarely in practice, untainted by "identity"). But this dip into the past leads us to ask another, less convenient question of our moment: If identitarian politics enabled a radicalism of which current theoretical postulations are rarely capable, can we really purchase so much utopian good by disavowing (as opposed to diversifying and expanding) them?

The current critical disdain for the identitarian participates in tendencies Judith Halberstam has astutely critiqued in her observation that the queer emphasis on performatively "flexible desires/practices/identifications marks people with strong identifications as pathological in relation to their rigidity and . . . the binary of flexible and rigid is definitely a temporal one — it ascribes mobility over time to some notion of liberation and creates stubborn identification as a way of being stuck in time, unevolved, not versatile" ("Theorizing Queer Temporalities," 190). Yet despite her critical sensitivity to rhetoric that belittles the past, Halberstam's own *In a Queer Time and Place* theorizes the "queer time" experienced during the age of AIDS without reference to the past. "The constantly diminishing future creates a new emphasis on the here, the present, the now" (2), Halberstam reports, situating the present *as* the past in a way that allows no room for the possibility that the past could live through memory *as* the present. The idea of the past is relegated to a category titled "Future Histories," which justifies the work of documenting the present as establishing an "archive" that may "become an important resource later for future queer historians who want to interpret the lives we have lived from the few records we have left behind" (45–46). In this model of the queer past, the clock starts now: there is a present that will become history in the future but no past worth recalling as a realm of possibility in the present and, by extension, the future.

Recent theorizations of "queer space," which insist on the unmarked performativity of a stealthy public sexual life that leaves no traces, similarly render unthinkable the idea that spatial signs might transmit past experience into the present. This exclusive focus on unmarked spatiality precludes the conceptual possibility that a space might retain its experiential markings. As we show in chapter 2, "For Time Immemorial: Marking Time in the Built Environment," this possibility was made manifest in AIDS memorials, public sex graffiti, and eventually in state-sanctioned public monuments.

Well-founded critiques of reproductive and generational futurity, aimed at hollow promises of payoff at a never-specified day-to-come for good behavior in the present rendered many academics in the late 1980s and since skeptical of *any* claims for transformation, even (often especially) those put forward by early gay or feminist liberationists.[8] The so-called antisocial turn in queer theory, initiated by Leo Bersani, maintained some of the confrontational and erotic spirit of criticism in the era of the sexual revolution but shifted ideas about agency from historically situated collectivity to psychically produced individualism or decorporealization. Frequently recasting street activism and public sex cultures accompanied by exuberant hopefulness and joyous pleasure as psychic disruption and unmanageable *jouissance,* first-wave queer theorists turned the depression and anxiety generated by AIDS and neoconservativism into dehistoricized forces of shame and other death-driven affects, positing these as the affective norm of queer life. While valuable and socially grounded theoretical work exploring psychic forces was done by theorists such as Eve Kosofsky Sedgwick, David Halperin, Judith Butler, and others, one consequence was to dehistoricize the queer psyche along with the socially located affects of shame, anxiety, and depression generated by the deaths, violence, and social stigma arising from AIDS. Resistances to acknowledging the historical contexts for the turn in the early 1990s to shame and psychic disaggregation made it significantly harder to identify with, and hence respond to, their historical as well as their psychic causes. As we argue in chapter 4, the dehistoricizing effect of much (although not all) psychoanalytic-based queer theory was to push out of critical view the hopeful affects and transformative agendas of an earlier generation, with the result that younger critics began calling for those very social and affective states *in the future,* making futurity the displaced location of the past. When critics did look backward, it was often to critique the beliefs and cultural forms that made earlier cultural models possible (forms now often dismissed as "identity politics" or "homonormativity"). While the instantiations of these trends sometimes offer incisive analyses of queer textuality and culture, collectively they unwittingly participate in the unremembering begun by conservative forces with whom few queer theorists would willingly be allied.

In the wake of these assaults on and erosions of memory from the left and the right, unremembering became the order of the day. It might be argued that gays, by the opening years of the millennium, had a lot to forget. Individual stories of unhappiness abounded; antigay violence and legislative setbacks were common; the collective trauma of AIDS was a fact of life. Just when we most needed models of culture that would allow us to mourn our losses and strengthen ourselves to resist the conservatism that made those losses seem inevitable, just when our pleasures and the cultural spaces for enjoying them were most precarious, we began a process of temporal isolation, distancing ourselves from the supposedly excessive generational past in exchange for promises of "acceptance" in mainstream institutions. The signs of these losses are everywhere: in the monopoly of "gay marriage" in place of debates about sexual world-making; in the assimilation of sexual minorities and the subsequent abandonment of supposedly restrictive gay "ghettos"; in the insistent invisibility of AIDS or sexual liberation in popular media; in the dearth of radical, public, and collective challenges to mainstream institutions. When young Americans today say that sexuality "just doesn't matter," it is often heralded as a progressive triumph. But sexuality *should* matter: it should be the thrilling, dangerous, unpredictable, imaginative force it once was and no doubt still is, although more often quietly and out of public sight. If sexuality does not matter anymore, it is not because we won but because of how much we have lost.

The sweeping calls to unremember targeted the generation hardest hit by the onset of AIDS, cutting that generation off from younger gays and lesbians who might continue the visionary work undertaken in the late 1960s and 1970s. We call this temporal isolation *de-generation*. It is a process destructive of both a generation of social revolutionaries and the transgenerational bonds that make the transmission of revolutionary projects and cultures across and against time possible. De-generational unremembering is not simply an assault on the past or an attempt at prophylactic protection of the future, then; it is, above all, an aggressive assault on possibilities for the queer present.

We call the phenomenon of distancing the past "unremembering" for two reasons. Above all, the act of distancing the past is a perpetual process, not a once-and-for-all forgetting. The end result is not, as was claimed by its neoconservative advocates, a prophylactic erasure of connections with the past but rather a perpetual self-monitoring for inclinations to pastness. Like Lot's wife, we are urged never to cast our eyes back, never to turn from a dubious vision of normativity-as-progress glimmering beyond a perpetually receding horizon. Rather than deferring satisfaction to a goal of achieving institutionalized normativity in the future, however, we want to advocate strategic remembering. Or—to put things in the unashamedly campy terms associated with earlier generations—looking for happiness, like Dorothy Gale, in our own backyards. This book is an effort to exploit the inventive and idealistic operations of memory in order to use recollections of exercises of freedom pioneered by previous gay generations to create a collective connection with the past that enables us as we transform the present. We intend this remembering to challenge the disciplines imposed upon—and often internalized within—gay culture. For what are disciplined in calls for unremembering are not traces of past sexual practices carried into the present (those were already done in by the shock of the epidemic's onslaught),[9] but rather a recuperative longing with the potential to *exceed* the inventive idealism of the past in the guise of remembering what took place in previous generations. That yearning in the guise of memory cannot be suppressed once and for all: it requires continual monitoring and self-correction, giving "unremembering" the perpetual life of the gerund.

The other reason we choose "unremembering" to describe an only partially achieved forgetting has to do with the forms of temporal distancing that have accompanied the traumatic losses occasioned by AIDS and by the policed conservatism that followed on the heels of those losses. Trauma causes an incomplete eradication: the traumatic experience hovers, not forgotten but not remembered, on the edge of consciousness. Among the historical disasters addressed by trauma theory (the Holocaust, the Vietnam War, 9/11), AIDS has rarely been taken up as one of the most significant cultural traumas of the late twentieth century, and the cultural aftershocks of reinvigorated assaults on gay lifeways has attracted even less attention as a site of trauma worthy of study.[10] Our hope here is to make de-generational unremembering visible as a traumatic cycle in which the violence of loss triggers a traumatic turning-away that, only half accomplished, perpetuates trauma through near-forgettings of a past that was a site not only of trauma but of pleasure and aspiration as well.

Remembering the "sexual revolution," we suggest, offers models for critiquing and creating pleasurable alternatives to the normative and traumatized present. Beyond the need to remember something specific, however, we claim that memory is an act of resistance, regardless of its content. By "memory" we mean a process at once disruptive and inventive. While memories are conventionally assumed to be relatively transparent retrievals of directly experienced pasts, we understand memory differently. Recent psychological studies have shown that memories are strongly influenced by subsequent events, which have the capability not only of highlighting experiences that seemed insignificant at the time but even — and quite often — of fabricating what seem to be memories out of a need for them to be true.[11] Such creativity within memory is not pernicious but rather is the way humans order the world to achieve a sense of coherence and meaning. Without getting into the scientific debates about the extent and mechanisms of memory construction, we accept the central argument that memories are not retrievals of an archived past but something more imaginative and more driven by present needs. It's not that memories have *no* relation to experience — they may, but they may not, or may do so only partially. It is the creative aspect of memory that makes it valuable as a socially transformative medium. Memories may come, as it were, third hand, from mass media or elite culture, from others' recollections, from another period's visual or print traces, from conjecture based on observation in the present. The fundamental point we stress is that memory is produced from need: singly or collectively, we remember what we need to know.

In focusing primarily on memory narratives that have taken aesthetic form (films, art installations, television shows, novels, monuments), we mean to foreground the creative and audience-directed nature of memory. Readers will doubtless recognize that many (if not most) of the memory narratives discussed in the following chapters are idealized, inaccurate (by the judgment of other people's recollected experience), anachronistic, or even invented. Such criticisms are beside the point. If memories were simply relived experience, they would be valueless for the present. Because memories are answerable to the needs of the present, they are shaped in relation to changed and changing social conditions. To take just one example from the memory narratives we examine, condoms have a symbolic significance they probably would not have had in the remembered time. Such memories respond to the intervening advent of ideas of "sexual responsibility" as a consequence of AIDS. Memories may also be corrective, envisioning multiethnic queer communities including men and women in ways that do not necessarily represent the experience of those who lived in those communities (while other memory narratives that we discuss in the first chapter, such as Marlon Riggs's *Tongues Untied*, address those exclusions head on, or such as Gus Van Sant's *Milk*, quote previous memory narratives, generating what we might think of as *meta*memories). We see these adaptations not as failures — as false memories — but as the core of *all* memories, which are always constructed and citational in ways that meet the needs of the present.

Memories enable more than survival; they are imaginative ways to disrupt and transform conditions that make survival necessary. Like utopias, memories craft a world that stands as a counterreality to the lacking or painful present, creating narratives of "the past" so as to challenge the inevitability of dominant constructions of "reality." The space-off and time-out of memory afford a critical distance from which to evaluate present conditions that lead to alienation and yearning as we picture alternatives that challenge the inevitability of those conditions and imagine other social arrangements that transform "reality" into a more livable (relation to) time and place.

In layering the seemingly inevitable *now* with creative alternatives, memory moves the present sideways, in the ways that Kathryn Bond Stockton has described queer children "growing sideways" rather than "growing up" into mature heterosexuality. Queer childhood, for Stockton, partakes "of the horizontal — what spreads sideways — or sideways and backwards — more than a simple thrust toward height and forward time" (*The Queer Child*, 4). The queer child is, for Stockton, a spectral presence, someone "who we are not and, in fact, never were" but who takes on a powerfully ghostly shape "by looking back" in our "unreachable fancy, making us wonder" (5). Far from being signs of loss, the spectral past becomes, for Stockton, a way to "fatten" the present, to move it sideways — even backward. If we think of queer culture as having a spectral childhood, a collective past, Stockton helps us see how our memories enlarge the present, suffusing it with "energy, pleasure, vitality, and (e)motion" that come through memory's "back-and-forth" (13) movements.

In rendering the present "fat" through its sideways (and backward) movements, memory responds to what Eve Kosofsky Sedgwick names the "desire of a reparative impulse" that is "additive and accretive" ("Paranoid Reading," 27–28). The fear that often accompanies reparative desire, Sedgwick writes, "is that the culture surrounding it is inadequate or inimical to its nurture" (28). Despite this fear, the reparative impulse "wants to assemble and confer plenitude on an object that will then have resources to offer to an inchoate self" (28). In the following chapters, memory is reparative in just this sense: its turn to the past signals the inadequacy of a present incapable (and unwilling) to nurture challenging social imaginings; its enhancement comprises a creative statement of yearning; its combination of past, present, and future generates the plenitude made possible by accretion; and its articulation of a different version of reality provides resources for an "inchoate self" that is collective as well as individual. A culture, that is, can be reparative in its collective memories, its desire being to repair the present rather than faithfully to restore the past. In naming "camp" as one such culturally reparative practice, Sedgwick notes its "prodigal production of alternative historiographies" and its "hilarious antiquarianism" (28). Sedgwick's description of camp suggests that the desire for reparation has always sought satisfactions in the past, where it reconfigures not only what has been lost but the very structures of remembering ("prodigal historiographies") as well. The cultural memories we explore in the following chapters are often campy and always imaginatively retrospective. That they are suffused with hope and determination as well as fear has everything to do with their being cast not in the future but in the past, a site not (only) of loss but also of reparative plenitude.

What allows memory to continue producing plenitude in the face of fear (of loss, of disbelief, of disappointment) is precisely its *pastness*. As we show in chapter 5, "Remembering a New Queer Politics: Ideals in the Aftermath of Identity," the pastness of memories, rather than any empirical truthfulness, gives vision the force of possibility. Asserting the *once having been* status of memory's content, its previous existence as a socially viable reality (whether or not that "real" ever existed), the pastness of memory forestalls claims that such alternative versions of reality *could*

not be. Unlike utopias, which cast their visions into a perpetually receding future, prone to dismissal on the grounds of implausibility, memories insist that what once was might be again. With the asserted pastness
of memory comes responsibility (and empowerment) to imagine material forms for unimaginable realities, aesthetically transforming the past,
as have the artists, writers, and filmmakers we discuss in the following
chapters, so as to transform the present. That is the imaginatively reparative work of memory.

Memory's Time

Although its assertion of pastness might seem to reinforce concepts of
chronological time, memories perform their work by refusing the dis-
crete borders of sequential "moments" and by collapsing the past and the
future into the present. Invoking a flawed present that relies on the past
for reparation, memories resist the notion of time moving progressively
to the step of constant betterment. The past, in memory, augments the
present and proposes templates for the future. Progressive time presumes
and supports logics of disciplined labor and of reproduction and development, logics that prioritize the generational futurity exemplified by
children and mark queers as stuck in a traumatized "phase." Memory's
collapse of chronological, progressive time, therefore, is one of its most
potent features. It is also the feature that has made memory a preoccupation for philosophers and theorists from John Locke to E. P. Thompson
and contemporary theorists of queer temporality, all of whom advocate
for memorial connections with the spectral past as a way to imagine more
viable social models in the present.

The section "On Retention" in John Locke's treatise *An Essay concerning Human Understanding* (first published in 1690) describes memory
as "the power to revive again, in our Minds those Ideas, which after im-
printing have disappeared, or have been as it were laid aside out of Sight"
(75). Memory becomes especially important for Locke in relation to ideas,
which appear as the surplus of quotidian reality that supplies the repeti-
tive rituals that turn "ideas" into lived experience. Socially abject ("laid
aside out of sight") as reality's other, ideas, Locke argues, "if they be not
sometimes renewed by repeated Exercise of the Senses, or Reflection"
disappear "and at last there remains nothing to be seen" (76). Forgetting

and mortality are rhetorically linked for Locke, who describes the act of forgetting as a deadly encryption/inscription. "Thus the *Ideas,*" he writes, "as well as Children, of our Youth, often die before us: And our Minds represent to us those Tombs, to which we are approaching; where though the Brass and Marble remain, yet the Inscriptions are effaced by time, and the Imagery moulders away" (76–77). The tomb of forgetfulness can be exhumed, however, and the accumulation of abject sensations Locke calls "ideas" returned to social viability, with the aid of passion. Given his association of encryption and inscription, it's tempting to read this exhumation as a propulsion of passionate ideas beyond scripted conventions into an antinomian realm of possibility. As Locke notes, near-forgotten ideas are "very often roused and tumbled out of these dark Cells, into open Day-light, by some turbulent and tempestuous Passion" (77).

For our purposes, there are several queer features of memory as set forth by Locke. First, for Locke memory is a struggle over corporeality: to forget is not simply to lose a thought or image; it is to lose the accumulation of *sensation,* and hence to lose the experiential life of the body itself. In this sense, memory takes on a simultaneously somatic and salvific capacity to retain life after the body that experiences has passed chronologically beyond the moment of memory. Second, Locke saw "passion" as essential to the resuscitation of life by memory, although we might reverse Locke's formulation and suggest that, while for Locke passion has an agency that precedes the return of memory, it is equally possible that passion may be an *effect* of memory: that passionate sensations — the deepest "ideas," Locke asserts, are those associated with pleasure and pain — may *generate,* and not simply be retrieved by, present-day passion in the form of "turbulent and tempestuous" memories.

In addition to entertaining the possibility of memory as generative of passion, we must move beyond the individual memories described by Locke in order to imagine a collective memory generative of social as well as sexual (social *and* sexual) pleasures. Locke's tomb may issue forth individual bodies, but he begins his description of that process with the image of dead children. The plural occupation of the tomb of forgetting is thus an image not only for the infantile, which is so often associated with gay sexuality, but for the imaginative sociality that is the latent object of forgetting over which Locke mourns. He returns to this idea of memory-as-sociality later in the *Essay.* "Ideas lodg'd in the memory," Locke writes, are "revived in the Mind," which "takes notice of them, as of a former Impression, and renews its acquaintance with them, as with Ideas it had known before. So that though *Ideas* formerly imprinted are not all constantly in view, yet in remembrance they are constantly known to be such" (77). Locke's shift from the singular "impression" to the plural "ideas" is significant, for the forms brought forth by memory are like acquaintances who, though they may appear sequentially, in fact exist simultaneously, something like a crowd. Sociality thus subverts (and is in turn enabled by) the sequential temporality that necessarily supplants the past with the present and that helps inscribe progressive narratives of maturity that might well result, as they do in Locke's description, in dead children.

It may be this resistance to the temporal sequencing, central to narratives, that leads Locke, like David Hume after him, to describe memory as an image rather than a story. Beyond the inscribed brass and marble "impressions" on the crypts of forgetfulness, Locke describes memory as a painting. Because sensations are *"drawn in our Minds"* in *"fading Colours,"* Locke contends, they require passionate memory for restoration; "if not sometimes refreshed," Locke warns, the colors of memory will "vanish and disappear" (76–77). It seems significant in this regard that many of the memories we examine here come not in texts but in visual culture: film and video, street furniture, sculpture. Given Locke's imagery, memory might be said to be the proper domain of the visual in an age when both maturity and progress are ordered by the supplanting sequencing of narrative temporality.

It is tempting as well to speculate that, on the threshold of the great age of mobility, when unprecedented numbers of people left behind families and communities in which they were known in order to enter the relative anonymity of cities, memory might have taken on an added importance, particularly in reference to "acquaintances." In the city, such spectral acquaintances might be the source of reviving passions, linking collectivity and passion in memory. Locke's theory of memory brings to mind the flâneur, an early queer figure whose strolls through the urban landscape proved both pleasurable and, from the perspective of progressive time, wasteful.

The importance of wasting time queerly becomes clear in E. P. Thompson's landmark 1968 essay, "Time, Work-Discipline, and Industrial Capitalism," which maps the changes that industrial capitalism brought to conceptions of time and labor. Where preindustrial economies were based on what Thompson calls "task-orientation"—a system of labor in which effort is expended in relation to the demands of specific tasks following natural cycles—industrial capitalism, he argues, generated "new disciplines, new incentives, and a new human nature upon which these incentives could bite effectively" (57). Industrialism's "intricate subdivision of processes" necessitated a "synchronization of labor" (70) that relied on regimes of "bells and clocks" and the disciplinary apparatus of "the supervision of labour; fines; . . . money incentives; preachings and schoolings; the suppression of fairs and sports" (90). Through these regimes, "new labour habits were formed, and a new time-discipline was impressed" (90), generating "a clear distinction between 'work' and 'life'" (93). Thompson locates this "new human nature," organized in relation to clock time, in a range of institutional disciplines, including religion (Thompson traces this process from Puritanism to its culmination in the aptly named Methodism) and education (school regimes organized by the clock prepared subjects for the temporal logic of industrialism). "Puritanism," Thompson writes, "in its marriage of convenience with industrial capitalism, was the agent which converted men to new valuations of time; which taught children even in their infancy to improve each shining hour; and which saturated men's minds with the equation, time is money" (95).

As Thompson notes, however, new time-disciplines did not change human nature without a fight. Because workers familiar with task-orientation resisted the changes brought by industrialism, time-discipline advanced in the name not only of productive labor but of good character and moral well-being. Thompson quotes the *Law Book of the Crowley Iron Works,* which justified its 100,000-plus words of rules and regulations as dedicated to "the end that sloath and villany should be detected and the just and diligent rewarded." To that end, pay was calculated to exclude time spent "being at taverns, alehouses, coffee houses, breakfast, dinner, playing, sleeping, smoaking, singing, reading of news history, quarrelling, contention, disputes or . . . any way loytering" (81). Those who wasted time in such unproductive ways found themselves targets of evangelical reform, as idleness became an affront to morality as well as to productive labor. These reform efforts, Thompson argues, targeted sociabilities enabled by "a vigorous and licensed popular culture" that had emerged during the early stages of industrialism and which "the propagandists of discipline regarded with dismay" (80). What were being "reformed," in other words, were collective forms of nonproductive pleasure, which, "flouting the urgency of respectable time-values" (95), made time itself "a place of the most far-reaching conflict" (93).

Although Thompson takes no account of sexuality (despite his use of metaphors such as "marriage of convenience") in this persuasive account, the traits he identifies as flouting time-disciplines — idleness, excessive appetite, self-indulgence, disputation, mobility across socially separated groups — had already become, at industrialism's inception, associated with sex, which more than any social vice was depicted as resistant to (re)productive time.[12] In the fiction of the late eighteenth and early nineteenth centuries, for instance, sexualized figures — libertines, seducers, wanton women, lascivious schoolteachers, prostitutes, rapacious men of the cloth, insatiable slaves and other people of color — not only wasted their own time but seduced others into wasting theirs as well.[13] These figures were particularly dangerous when they operated, as they often did, within the institutions central to the internalization of time-discipline, especially churches and schools, or when they emerged from a bygone day and its outmoded economic system, such as bankrupted aristocrats or the sons and daughters of ruined rural farmers and merchants. At home only in the past, such characters are often nostalgic, seeking (hopelessly, the novels suggest) to recapture either the luxury or innocence of an economy that has disappeared. Caught "out of time," these sexualized characters, far from being well-paced and orderly, are frantically ad hoc, engaging in a sexualized version of task-orientation as they set out to seduce maidens, escape jealous spouses, hide pregnancies, find their next monetary dupe. To be sexual is, in the logic of these novels, to be lost in time, which is in turn to be disastrously ruined.

Moving from fictional societies to social fictions, these countertemporal traits — nostalgia, self-indulgence, insatiable desire, unproductive frivolousness — were by the end of the nineteenth century consolidated into the newly emerged figure of the dandy, a figure of gender ambiguity and sexual excess, who became under the influence of Oscar Wilde's trials inextricably identified as homosexual.[14] "It is only the Philistine who seeks to estimate a personality by the vulgar test of Production," Wilde wrote in "Pen, Pencil and Poison," his provocative encomium to the artist, essayist, forger, and murderer Thomas Griffiths Wainewright, adding, "This young dandy sought to be somebody, rather than to do something" (*Intentions*, 65). The fops of Wilde's essays and plays are all prodigious time wasters. One might argue that the "homosexual," as an identity defined by unproductive expenditures of time as much as by unproductive sex acts, is the embodiment of decades of reformist stereotypes aimed at naturalizing and implanting the time-disciplines of the industrial West. As such, "homosexuality" is also the name of a received history of resistance to those disciplines of orderly and progressive time, perhaps of time itself. Always running out of time, homosexuals stand in for all those who looked backward, yearning for different erotic ethics located in another time, located more in fantasy than in fact. When the nineteenth-century aesthete Walter Pater quoted the eighteenth-century art historian Johann Winckelmann in an essay now often cited as a foundational document of modern "homosexual" identity, the phrase he hit upon was, "I have come into the world and into Italy too late" (*Studies in the Renaissance*, 189). Nostalgic longing arising from a temporal disorientation in the present was thus central to the emergence of modern homosexual identity. Within and beyond this nineteenth-century inception, homosexuals have been principal representatives and agents of memory, which we conceive, following that representational tradition, as an imaginative restaging of now-proscribed sexual ethics as a past "reality" that, having once existed, might exist again as a differently temporalized, vastly more eroticized and nonproductive present.

Given the history of sexuality's relation to contests over time and productivity, a relation dating back to the inception of industrial capital, it is no surprise that contested conceptions of time and sexuality emerged again as nation-states, which during the Cold War became the rationale for industrial discipline and guaranteed its status as "freedom," lost their hold on the global economy. During the Cold War, the Soviet Union was a powerful external threat to capitalism, likened in the political rhetoric of the period to homosexuals who were often equated with communist sympathizers as powerful agents of corruption from within. The end of the Cold War in the 1980s threatened the dominance of the associated "military industrial complex," as the economy of the United States gravitated toward services that could, with the development of Internet technology, be located away from a central workplace and its temporal orders and as industrial labor was "outsourced" to Third World countries, challenging the centrality of the nation-state. In the face of these challenges to nationalism and the militarized industry it rationalized, politicians in the United States (and their imitators in Great Britain) scrambled to find new "alien" enemies, generating panics that eventually focused on illegal immigrants and religious terrorists. Politicians also regenerated an "enemy within," gays and lesbians. Just as the Cold War needed an internal threat to supplement its external one, so the new political order found its "other," as it had in the previous century, in the sexually "deviant." As home-labor threatened to erode the disciplinary lines between public and private life, new panics over sexual predation in public spaces, schools, and over the Internet, redrew those lines by prescribing the defensive separation of a secure "home" and a malicious "world." Anxieties over changing gender roles and sexual norms consolidated into concerted campaigns of homophobia, which became more violent as simultaneously the Cold War concluded and the AIDS epidemic began. Gays and lesbians were cast as a threat against which "family values" and the institution of marriage had to be protected. With AIDS, the counterprogressive traits associated with homosexuality — nostalgia for times past and indulgence in the sexual nonreproductivity of pleasure, which refuses a future figured as "our children's children" — were cast as threats not only to individual homosexuals or the economic structure they opposed but to the survival of humanity.

The redisciplining of queer life took hold in the gay community itself in the form of "forward-looking" rights activism centered on gaining gay men and lesbians entrance into two of the prime modern institutions of time-discipline: the family (conceived in terms of monogamous and reproductive couple-based marriage) and the military. This shift was countered, as the following chapters discuss, by queer cultural activism across a range of media that insisted on memory and its relation to sexual pleasure and social diversity. Many, if not all, of these temporal skirmishes began with the AIDS epidemic and its cultural effects, but they open onto issues central to understanding the threatened demise of a nation-based economic and industrial order.

At the end of his essay, Thompson speculates about the possibility that "if the purposive notation of time-use becomes less compulsive," then "men might have to re-learn some of the arts of living lost in the industrial revolution: how to fill the interstices of their days with enriched, more leisurely, personal and social relations" ("Time, Work-Discipline," 95). Memories, particularly those of the broad array of ideals and initiatives encapsulated under the rubric of "the sexual revolution," do precisely this: they look backward to forms of popular culture that worked against time-discipline in order to enhance the pleasures of leisure and the inventive socialities they enabled. It's not coincidental that when in 1974 Charley Shively talked about "promiscuity" as a revolutionary act, he conceived this rebellion as countering the strict separation of leisure and productive labor that, according to Thompson, was the result of time-discipline. If promiscuity were available everywhere, not just in the bedroom, Shively argued, work would not be drained of its vitality nor would pleasure be isolated to a very small time spent in the bedroom. The breakdown of the divide between private and business life, in Shively's account, would produce what he called a sexual socialism: greater opportunities for human development and equitable sociability across lines of rank, color, or privilege. In arguing that we should remember earlier theorists of sexuality like Shively, as we do in chapter 4, we contend that such memories would provide and enable better models for sexual sociability (and for sociability generally) at a moment when the time-disciplines analyzed by Thompson are once again up for grabs.

We cannot, of course, simply return to an earlier era in sexual culture, for, as Thompson cautions, "no culture re-appears in the same form" at a later time (96). Yet there is value in looking back, even if the views afforded by backward glances remain beyond reclaiming. Cultural dissidents at earlier stages of industrial capitalism were also backward-looking in, for example, the fantasies of ancient Greece and Rome that characterized Victorian sexual dissidents like Pater and Wilde; Edward Carpenter's 1906 *Ioläus* is a catalog of references to erotic intimacy between men throughout history and around the world. These reformers did not propose that paradigms from the past could simply be reinhabited but rather cited the alternative socialities of other times and other places to prove that different social models once existed and might, therefore, become social reality again. In their temporal turns backward, dissenters refused the productive orders of time-discipline and thereby kept open the possibility not of reclamation but of reparation in the present. At the end of time-discipline, Thompson conjectures, what will emerge is not an integral past but "a new synthesis" combining "elements of the old and of the new, finding an imagery based neither upon the seasons nor upon the market but upon human occasions. . . . And unpurposive passing of time would be behaviour which the culture approved" (96). We see memory as just such an act of synthesis, a way imaginatively to summon other systems of social organization and pleasure, not as importations from the past but as a use of pastness to articulate social yearnings that contest the disciplines of the present.

Bringing together Thompson's analysis of a time-discipline resisted by alternative sociabilities with Locke's understanding of how the passionate enactment of memory revitalizes a mortifying present, we come to something like the theory of memory as performance offered by Tavia Nyong'o. Seeing memory "as a collective and participatory phenomenon occurring within 'the social frameworks of memory,'" Nyong'o contends that the performance of memory, "as restored or 'twice behaved' behavior mediates between collective memory and the new, potential, and virtual" (*The Amalgamation Waltz,* 13). The potential generated by performed memory, in Nyong'o's analysis, cracks open the "realist form upon which both the nation-state and its fantasy of homogenous, empty time rest." In place of "a time of training, waiting, and indefinite deferral," of "life lived in the antechamber of history" (12), Nyong'o proposes performative time, which "seize[s] upon national narratives with a disruptive immediacy" and is "filled with the presence of the now and that thereby call[s] the bluff of the ruse of postponement" (12).

These accounts tell us much about memory's usefulness in disrupting the coerced temporalities of industrialism and the nation-state, about its capacity to imagine and perform new social relations in a context of passion, and about how the past becomes a site of resistance and reparation in the here and now. They show us, in short, why memory is so queer. Not surprisingly, several contemporary theorists have analyzed memory and temporality explicitly as a mode of queer world-making, heeding Christopher Nealon's call "to understand, through an identification with an ancestor, how history works, what it looks like, what possibilities it has offered in the past, and what those possibilities suggest about our ineffable present tense" (*Foundlings,* 86).

Taking up this call, theorists have underscored queer temporality's power to resist progressive, chronological time, or what Dana Luciano calls "national time," and to refill what Walter Benjamin called "homogenous empty time" with reparative plenitude. Elizabeth Freeman describes how memory becomes "a means of addressing history in an idiom of plea-

sure," and she observes the frequency with which "perverts — melancholi-
cally attached to obsolete erotic objects or fetishes they ought to have out-
grown, or repeating unproductive bodily behaviors over and over — refuse
the commodity-time of speedy manufacture and planned obsolescence"
("Turn the Beat Around," 34–35). Freeman argues that memory becomes
for queers a potent form of social critique that uses "physical sensation to
break apart the present into fragments of time that may not be one's 'own'
or to feel one's present world as both conditioned and contingent" (38).
Carla Freccero writes of a "queer spectrality" that serves "as a phantasmatic relation to historicity that could account for the affective force of
the past in the present, of a desire issuing from another time and placing
a demand on the present in the form of an ethical imperative" ("Theorizing Queer Temporalities," 184) Working through, in Freeman's words,
"retrogression, delay, and the pull of the past upon the present" ("Packing
History, Count(er)ing Generations," 728), queer memory, comprising the
pleasurable disorder and the visualized possibilities Locke and Thompson
found in memory, generates what Nealon describes as "huddled temporalities, allergic to the present tense" (*Foundlings,* 180).

The queer ability to bond affectively with the past is particularly important, Ann Cvetkovich argues, in "the absence of institutional documenta-
tion or in opposition to official histories," making memory "a valuable historical resource, and ephemeral and personal collections of objects stand
alongside the documents of the dominant culture in order to offer alternative modes of knowledge" (*An Archive of Feelings,* 8). While Cvetkovich
imagines an archival memory documenting the lived past, there are important distinctions to be drawn between memory and history. Memory
is a broader category than history, not only because it allows for the archiving of acts, affects, and attitudes often denied the status of historical
record but because it is incomplete, fragmented, affect-saturated, and for
these reasons continually open to the imaginative processes of rearticula-
tion, reinvention, and adaptation. Virginia Woolf's recollection of Judith
Shakespeare, William's imagined-as-forgotten sister, stands as a powerful paradigm for acts of memory beyond the archive. Sitting uneasily on
the borders of public and private, individual and collective, historical and
ephemeral, desire and impression, memory takes up the detritus of loss
and preserves it more as a strategic, pliable, and evanescent expression
than as a fixed monument or accurate rendition.

Pliable time, as Locke well understood, produces alternative sociality. Just as past ideas, for Locke, become regained acquaintances, so, for queer theorists like Carolyn Dinshaw, "queer historical touches" help "form communities across time." Such communities, forged through "the funny communicability of shadow-relations and secret emotions," form communities with the future as well as the past and project more pleasurable, inclusive, and just social relations *as* the queer future ("Theorizing Queer Temporalities," 178). Encouraging us to consider sexuality itself "as a model of address, as a set of relations, lived and imagined, that are perpetually cast out ahead of our 'real,'" Nealon proposes an "imagined community" rooted not in identities but in ideals that take us both backward and forward, envisioning future social pleasures that we share with figures from the past (*Foundlings*, 180). Complicating "the idea of horizontal political generations succeeding one another with a notion of 'temporal drag,'" Freeman notes, queer temporality, especially in the form of memory, replaces "the psychic time of the individual" with "the movement time of collective political life" ("Packing History, Count(er)ing Generations," 729). Because of this, "memory can prop up projects unrelated to the history it supposedly preserves" as it reconfigures the possible by adding "a codicil of pleasure to a legacy of suffering" ("Turn the Beat Around," 55, 63).

The only temporal phenomenon these queer theories do not address is their own engagement with questions of time and memory. Ironically, much queer temporal theory, in formulating the deep communities of feeling between past and present, performatively *dis*connects theory from history by ignoring the relationship of its concerns to the social specificities of its present, particularly the temporal warps brought about by AIDS, or to the theoretical and social insights of the past that might help us respond to cultural reactions to the epidemic. Ann Cvetkovich is an exception, poignantly acknowledging that her "desire, forged from the urgency of death, has been to keep the history of AIDS activism alive and part of the present" (*An Archive of Feelings*, 6). Similarly, José Muñoz addresses "a primary relation to emotions, queer memories, and structures of feeling that haunt gay men on both sides of the generational divide that is formed by and through the catastrophe of AIDS" (*Cruising Utopia*, 41). Queer memory, for Muñoz, points "beyond the painful barriers of the AIDS pandemic" through "a certain conjuring of 'the past'" (38). Writing of the pre-AIDS "culture of sexual possibility" described by activist and critic Douglas Crimp, Muñoz concludes, "Although the moment that Crimp describes is a moment that is behind us, its memory, its ghosts, and the ritualized performances of transmitting its vision of utopia across generational divides still fuels and propels our political and erotic lives: it still nourishes the possibility of our current, actually existing gay lifeworld" (34).

In this spirit, we contend that AIDS has been a critical impetus for much academic work on queer time, including our own. The death of friends and the loss of generational transmission of cultural literacy, pleasures, and ideals threatened by those deaths and by phobic responses to them has moved us not only to remember but also to address the causes and consequences of not doing so. AIDS, devastating as it was, was not responsible for the unremembering that whittled the sexual revolution down to our current narrow options for politics and pleasure. As we show in the chapters that follow, other forces deployed prophylactic amnesia to produce the single-minded normative fixations that too often characterize sexual politics today. That story, we believe, is part of the powerful urgency of many, although not all, recent considerations of queer time and queer memory.[15]

Faced with the too-frequently disheartening history of AIDS and its cultural aftershocks, we have drawn from these critics a confirmation of memory's power to exhilarate and empower. We want, however, to acknowledge that although memory can help us create better presents, it cannot be expected to eliminate the sorrows and losses of the past, which must remain part of our memories. Memory is neither clean nor comforting, but is messy business, and never more so than when our efforts to "feel backward," as Heather Love persuasively demonstrates, produce ambivalence, uncertainty, and impatience alongside admiration, clarity, and joy. We must reckon with the past as well as reconcile and commune with it.

To acknowledge loss, however, is not to concede to the debilitating alienation that is conventionally assumed to characterize its survivors. Loss may be marked by silence and loneliness, bereavement and thwarted hopes. What is lost seems to vanish forever into an inarticulate void from which emerges nothing save the occasional memorial abstraction, fixed in the finite cast of a defeated ideal, rather than a living potential. To lose is to be translated into the victor's language, to become part of an eclipsed era, an ill-fated ambition, a relic in a display of what must not be tried again. Stunned and saddened, survivors scan their surroundings for any sign of a person loved, a world maintained, and find instead the victor's desires translated into the cheerful veneer of everyday life, uncontested, unconflicted, and ungrieved. But loss can be a powerful motivator too, and it has an important place in memory. Out of the losses due to AIDS, individual as well as collective, came a struggle over the legibility and meaning of the past, a struggle that, as we show in the following chapters, was always invested in social possibility in the present: the connectedness of interests beyond the enforced separations of identity; the emergence and continuous reinvention of alliances, pleasures, and signifying practices around the figure of sexed bodies and sexual cultures; the forging of a more generous, compassionate, and capacious understanding of what social bodies can make and maintain. While we are in sympathy with Muñoz's interest in "a force field of affect and political desire" that he calls *"queer utopian memory"* (*Cruising Utopia*, 35), we want to push beyond his concentration on remembrances of public sex that long "for a moment outside of this current state of siege" brought on by AIDS (47). We argue that the idealism associated with queer utopian memory need not operate outside loss but can function through and because of loss. As we argue throughout, the normalizing, de-generational insistence that we forget—that we cut ourselves off from the promise of the past and from those who bravely, smartly, imaginatively, naughtily, compassionately took up that promise—has never been completely heeded and obeyed. Rather it has challenged many of us to pay critical attention to what they tell us to forget and why, and to show how essential memory is to the articulation of queer subjects, queer subcultures, and progressive queer politics. Loss is not synonymous with silence or absence or defeat; loss can be a starting point, an invocation, an inspiration, a rallying cry. Necessity, it is said, is the mother of invention, and needs are never greater than in times of loss.

Remembering Whatever

In arguing for memory's reparative capabilities, we conceive of memory as a form of what Michel Foucault, in *The History of Sexuality,* called *askesis,* a meditative self-transformation central to the care of the self. But memory, as we've suggested, is also a collective practice, a *social askesis*, based not on identity or shared past experience but on a shared yearning (or different yearnings that find satisfaction in the same memory), including the yearning to belong. Memory enables what Foucault imagined in his late interviews as a transformative mode of relation, new social alliances and transformed ethics, predicated not on identity (although Foucault made particular claims for gay men's relation to memory) but on a common sense of the inadequacy of current relations and empirical ethics.[16] Looking for a way to care for selves, those engaged in memory creatively transform the present by looking to the past.

In order to understand the possible communities assembled through memory, it may be helpful to say what they are *not*. Specifically, they are not identity-based communities, even though their formative memories may involve identity-based content. Although the memory narratives examined here often focus on white gay men, for example, they comprise communities that are not necessarily white or gay or male. Identification, rather then identity, is central to memory, as we show in chapter 3, "The Revolution Might Be Televised: The Mass Mediation of Gay Memories," where we examine the chatrooms devoted to the television sitcom *Will and Grace*. The identification with white gay men in the 1970s by an unpredictable audience suggests to us that what participants (at least appreciative ones) in these memories share is not an identity but a desire, a shared sense of the inadequacy of the present. That these memories often transform historical record in order to accommodate the divergent (racial, gendered) identifications of those who remember is what makes memory a viable form of social protest and reparative imagining.

Communities formed through memory may be close to what Giorgio Agamben calls, in the title of his influential book, *The Coming Community*. Trying to locate *being* outside, on one hand, both universal generalities that make no allowance for deviations and, on the other, individualizing particularities that are part of no collectivity, Agamben focuses on the relationship between these conceptions, or what he calls *whatever* being. In a state of *whatever*, particularities become meaningful insofar as they can be contextualized in terms of a larger entity to which they are not reducible, and generalities take on meaning through an accumulation of particularities, which they fall short of fully naming. *Whatever* being becomes particularly suggestive when applied to people, who exist in relation to neither unique nor general ontology (individualism or humanity) but in the reaching of the former toward the latter, which Agamben calls *coming-to-being*. The state of coming-to-be is, for Agamben, saturated with possibility, since ontological surety is foreclosed and any assertion of *me*-ness would allow for the possibility of *not-me-ness*. The being open to not-being is what makes coming-to-being pure possibility, but it is also, Agamben claims, what makes ethics possible, since, unlike morals that have only one correct outcome, coming-to-being allows for multiple trajectories that must be ethically evaluated in relation to one another.

In the chapters that follow, memory functions as a mode of coming-to-being, of particular memories stretching toward a collective life balanced by the not-community of a lost past and a lacking present. The liminality of memory — poised between individuality and collectivity, presumed factuality and pure invention, past and future, loss and expectation — is what makes it *whatever*, a practice of ethical possibility in Agamben's sense, challenging the ontological, temporal, and moral certainties of the present's moral orders. Memories centered on gay sexual culture in the 1970s, for example, challenge the moral certainties of both the homophobic right and the rights-seeking left. Both groups, in demanding that rights be conferred on or withheld from gays, claim to know who gays "are," what legal outcomes that ontology justifies, and the moral trajectories (justice or immorality) that will arise, without possible detour, from granting or withholding rights. In opposition to such certainties, memory simultaneously considers modes of being and nonbeing (imagined communities lost to the past) in ways that are ethical rather than moral, open to multiple trajectories that are neither utopian (displaced to an imagined future) nor nostalgic (conceived as simply retrievable from the past). Agamben, in *The Coming Community*, imagines the halo that, in Catholic tradition, the dead receive on entering heaven as "a zone in which possibility and reality, potentiality and actuality, become indistinguishable" and in which the "being that has reached its end, that has consumed all its possibilities, thus receives as a gift a supplemental possibility" (56). If we translate Agamben's metaphysics into the quotidian work of remembering, we might say that memory, similarly located between the possible and the actual, reaches back to the (socially, temporally, mortally) dead to offer them a supplemental possibility in the minds of those who remember. Memory, in this sense, is the halo of the living.

The ethical state of being described by Agamben and carried out in memory does not rest with the individual subject but proposes alternative socialities. The reaching beyond particularity toward generality is motivated, after all, by a yearning to belong. But Agamben's coming community—like memory's—invokes a belonging with a difference. Just as *whatever* involves a simultaneous awareness of being and nonbeing, so belonging involves recognition of a belonging-outside, understood not as an anterior space but as "the experience of the limit itself, the experience of being-*within* an *outside*" (*The Coming Community*, 68). The being-within-an-outside takes on an ethical urgency in the face of contemporary politics, in which spectacles "take control of social memory and social control, transforming them into a single spectacular commodity where everything can be called into question except the spectacle itself" (80). Spectacles, for Agamben, dangerously alienate people from the possibility of what he calls "the Common," our capacity to belong without either ontological or moral certainty, an ethical being-within-an-outside. Expropriated from this ethical belonging, without "the very possibility of a common good" (80), we are prone to the destructive violence of spectacular politics. At the same time as it threatens violence, however, the spectacle also "retains something like a positive possibility that can be used against it" (80). Agamben does not linger on that "positive possibility," but we believe the performance of memory, particularly memories that arise from *within* commodity culture or mass media, represent just such a "positive possibility" within a politics of spectacle, expressing a desired belonging that goes beyond the confines of identity or moral certainty without surrendering ethical responsibility or what Agamben calls "the common good."

Understanding the radical potential of alternative temporalities, Agamben points to the reasons memory would become the means for imagining—and contesting—new forms of belonging. In *Infancy and History,* Agamben writes, "Every culture is first and foremost a particular experience of time, and no new culture is possible without an alteration of this experience. The original task of a genuine revolution, therefore, is never merely 'to change the world,' but also—and above all—to 'change time'" (99). Here Agamben argues for a need to revise a "vulgar representation of time as a precise and homogenous continuum" that divides "the present into discreet instants" (111). Against this concept of time, which Agamben calls "a fundamental sickness" that, "with its infinite postponement, hinders human existence from taking possession of itself as something full and singular," Agamben proposes the Stoics' concept of time as "neither objective nor removed from our control, but springing from the actions of man" (111).

For Agamben, the reversal of time is not an extraordinary occurrence but requires that one recognize the quotidian experience of what we might call "being-without-time." For everyone, he writes, "there is an immediate and available experience on which a new concept of time could be founded. This is an experience so essential to human beings that an ancient Western myth makes it humankind's original home: it is pleasure" (114). Far from being a frivolous pastime, pleasure is the experience and the content of a revolutionary pastime, or memory. "He who, in the epoch of pleasure, has remembered history as he would remember his original home, will bring this memory to everything, will exact this promise from each instant: he is the true revolutionary and the true seer, released from time not at the millennium, but *now*" (115). Memory thus leads Agamben not to a millennial utopianism but rather to the "now," in which the "original home," pleasure, is remembered so as to halt time and create a new present. The presence enabled by memory does not involve ontology, temporal or otherwise, then, but a present performance of a temporal displacement through memory that enables in turn what Muñoz calls "critical deployment of the past for the purpose of engaging the present" (*Cruising Utopia*, 116). Yet that engagement opens a space not (only) for "imagining the future" (116) but also for making new presents. If potentiality is our horizon (and we would agree that it is), it is a horizon seen only in the rearview mirror.

Being a collective without identity, the community imagined in and through memory may not be utopian but is nevertheless a provocation to the state, which, according to Agamben, cannot tolerate "that humans co-belong without any representable condition of belonging" (*The Coming Community*, 86). In the context of queer challenges to the state in the situation of AIDS and "moral majority" politics, it is little wonder that queer memory draws heat from all sides. While those seeking state recognition claim legitimacy purchased by a break with the sexual past, queer memory not only refuses to relinquish the past but makes pastness the core of resistant claims in defiance of legal acceptance. With both popular and elite culture taking up belongings enabled by memory, with historians deepening our understanding of past sexual cultures, with ACT UP and Queer Nation deploying that past to demand media attention in ways that took the power of spectacle from the state, memory became the field on which struggles over the meaning and possibilities of sexuality and belonging took place.

Remembering Amnesia; or, Dancing (Again) at Ground Zero

From this abstract consideration of memory, we return in closing to the embodied and the specific, in particular with regard to the memory content we take up in this book: gay culture during the "sexual revolution" of the 1970s and after. This is, in many ways, a book that could only have been written in middle age. In saying this, we refer both to our own middle age and to that of a cultural and political movement. When we were first coming out in the early 1980s at a small New England college in western Massachusetts, the "sexual revolution" was practically over, and what we knew of it came mostly from books such as Andrew Holleran's 1978 novel, *Dancer from the Dance,* which offered a taste of the music, sexual customs, and above all storytelling styles that flourished a mere 180 miles away in Manhattan. We now see that the novel told very little of the rich intellectual and political developments, discussed in chapter 4 here, that flourished alongside dance parties and sex publics. But it did depict a network of men in the city among whom — contrary to the plots of television soap operas both of the afternoon and evening variety in which ex-lovers are always the bitterest of enemies — sex led often to social ties rooted in trust, familiarity, and shared knowledge among men, even those who met briefly and never exchanged names. That knowledge was reinforced in the novel by a cultural vocabulary — deejays and dance divas, drugs, locations where men could find quick sex or night-long orgies, how to know who wanted "it" and which "it" he wanted — that showed how things the rest of the culture deemed trivial (or worse) could create a safe place in a hostile environment, a culture within a culture. The details of this culture's productive vocabulary changed quickly. It was not just promiscuous sex this culture was inventing; it was promiscuous representation. It was the nature of the things the culture valued — drugs, dance, music, cruising — to be constantly in flux, a dynamism that emphasized the apparent permanence of the network through which the details moved. Producing a rich culture in a world that considered them sick and immoral, the men in the novel could not count on archives and history books, but they could count on the communication networks generated through individual memory and, more important, through collectively circulated memory narratives.

By the time we moved to New York around 1982–83, the world depicted in Holleran's novel had largely vanished, giving the novel the feel of a *memento mori*. The world from which we had felt separated by geography now seemed to be put off limits temporally, turned, too literally, into a cultural skeleton in the closet. "'I don't know anyone who is gay anymore,' says a woman I know," Holleran reports in *Ground Zero*, his 1988 postmortem on the 1970s. "'Gay is not an option.' The bars, the discotheques that are still open seem pointless in a way; the social contract, the assumptions, that gave them their meaning, is gone [sic]" (21–22). Organizations were somber (the leader of the gay Marxist reading group in which one of us participated in 1984 committed suicide after his lover died from AIDS). Friends stopped going to bars and dances and started coupling up, feathering nests. If anyone still had tales of sexual adventure, he kept them to himself. The culture of *Dancer from the Dance* was disappearing because, as Holleran put it, sex had become "the Siamese twin of death" (*Ground Zero*, 20).

Holleran's metaphor of the Siamese twins makes the linkage of sex and death a natural phenomenon. The most powerful agent in the natural arsenal was, of course, the virus itself, which quickly took on anthropomorphic powers. "The death of Dionysus—the closing down of promiscuity—took a long time to complete itself," Holleran writes, "a lot of fear. But fear was what the plague has produced copiously, till it now constitutes the substance of homosexual life. AIDS has been a massive form of aversion therapy. For if you finally equate sex with death, you don't have to worry about observing safe sex techniques; sex itself will eventually become unappetizing" (24–25). Holleran's account of how sex got linked to death evacuates human agency and the forces of unremembering we outline in the following chapters in favor of the virus "itself." Given the high premium Holleran puts on narratives in the creation and perpetuation of sexual culture, however, it makes far more sense to attribute the eradication of that culture to human agents who worked to unremember rituals of memory and the narratives that sustain and are enabled by them. The death of the 1970s, the move from a cultural self-representation that valorized sexual adventure, expansion, and optimism to one that stressed harrowing guilt, isolation, and despair was neither a natural nor a historical inevitability but, as we argue throughout, the result of changes in representation that have had debilitating social and political consequences for sexual culture today.

Of course there was never the clean break between pre- and post-AIDS gay life that Holleran (and, in some ways, our own anthropomorphizing tale of gay culture) posits. Throughout the 1980s and 1990s, sexual culture continued despite police harassment, the closure of sex businesses, the "gentrification" of sex spaces, and the panic generated around sex acts themselves. As numerous critics have noted, ACT UP, formed in 1987, forged powerful connections between eroticism and politics, generating episodes of unprecedented political and culture power and representational ingenuity. Throughout this period, critics, artists, and historians such as Vito Russo, Douglas Crimp, Cindy Patton, Pat Califia, Marlon Riggs, Simon Watney, Sarah Schulman, Samuel Delany, David Wojnarowicz, John Boswell, Derek Jarman, Essex Hemphill, Dorothy Allison, George Chauncey, and Paula Treichler preserved the sexual "past" in archival history, dissident sexual practices, fierce critical analysis, and, most important for us, through a combination of outraged fury and hopeful idealism that characterized a previous generation of gay and lesbian culture. In the important 1987 essay "How to Have Promiscuity in an Epidemic," Douglas Crimp, a critic closely allied with ACT UP, writes, "All those who contend that gay male promiscuity is merely sexual *compulsion* resulting from fear of intimacy are now faced with very strong evidence against their prejudices. . . . Gay male promiscuity should be seen instead as a positive model of how sexual pleasures might be pursued by and granted to everyone if those pleasures were not confined within the narrow limits of institutionalized sexuality" (*Melancholia and Moralism,* 65). Because these activists kept the merging of pride, anger, community concern, compassion, tenderness, and exuberant fun thriving throughout the 1980s and 1990s, we can now reflect on a continuing, if changing, culture extending from the sexual revolution to the current day. Thinking through the transformative potential not of gay sex as much as of gay sexual culture, of gay promiscuous representation, these writers and artists demanded not only a place at the table, to borrow the title of Bruce Bawer's de-generational treatise, but a change of menu.

Even resisting the before-and-after narrative and acknowledging that human life spans fit uncomfortably on social movements, it became clear to us as we prepared this book, rereading, updating, and augmenting some of our previously published essays, that the arrangement of the chapters in this book itself constitutes a kind of memory, if not of "gay culture" writ large then at least of our own engagement with that culture. The first chapter, which confronts the initial push by gay neocons to unremember the sexual past, expresses the shock and anger that characterized the late 1980s and early 1990s, when most of the chapter was written. By the time the second chapter was written, a few years later, anger had largely given way to grief and a searching for a "homeland" that, by that time, was beginning to seem mortally, if not to say theoretically, elusive. Feeling like we were losing a community we relied on for the transmission of cultural memory, we were surprised to discover those memories in what might seem the unlikely venue of primetime television, a site we explore in our third chapter on the sitcom *Will and Grace* and the Internet chatrooms devoted to the show. By the time the fourth chapter was written, our attention was drawn to the institutionalization of queer theory in the academy. Here, too, we discovered battles over the meaning and usefulness of the sexual past, as we discuss in chapter 4, which involved characterizations of the past we sometimes could not reconcile with our own reading and experience. Finally, having lost identity politics to an academic critique in which the indubitable power of argument often seemed matched by a willful blindness to the ways that identity had enabled the academic forums in which the critique was articulated, we began to wonder what forms of belonging, if not identity based, might be possible in the aftermath of queer theory, of political constriction, and of AIDS. Our answer— "ideality politics"— became the subject of our final chapter.

While these chapters follow the ups and downs (and ups again) of social and emotional developments that were by no means ours particularly, we did make a conscious choice in our objects of study. In choosing those, we tried to take seriously E. P. Thompson's model of new social orders organized around "human occasions" that arise not from a pure place prior to or outside commodity capitalism but from syntheses that emerge through our experience of and with market economies. While we examine contests over memory as they occur in elite culture — the world of fine arts, indie film, avant-garde performance, and urban queer sub-culture — we also pay attention to the "popular culture" that, as Thompson notes, is where the debates over time-discipline emerged most dramatically. Rather than seeing television shows like *Will and Grace* as irredeemably corrupted by commodity culture or films like *Longtime Companion* as compromised by their mainstream distribution, we have taken these sites of memory seriously as productions of a temporal warp within American culture that has affected queer mass culture as well as elite culture and has, for that matter, transformed the commodity capitalism and mass distribution systems within which "the popular" circulates. We believe that, although beholden to commodity advertisement, mass culture is sometimes a vehicle for popular memory, bearing not only the allure of the commodity but also memories of other social pleasures and possibilities into the present. That these forms are available to significantly more people than are the productions of urban avant-gardes makes them all the more appealing to us as sites of creative memory and imaginative social reimagining. We also chose forms of popular culture that are materially present (public monuments, sculptures) and emotionally evocative (the sentimental or comic film) because we believe memory is the work not only of the conscious mind but of the somatic body as well.

In the spirit of memory in popular culture, we end by returning to the Memphis nightclub with which we began: recently, a posting paradoxically called "Remembering Amnesia" shared recollections about the now-closed club, ending with an announcement that another club, called Senses, would host a "Retro Amnesia Night." (Over)reading the names of nightclubs once more, we conclude that the closure(s) of amnesia can be at least partially undone by the persistence of sensual memory, which can invoke — without claiming to replicate — seemingly lost spaces and times "retro"-actively in the present. Joining those who came to (their) Senses, we too understand memory not as transparent or exact recovery but rather as an invitation to share memory narratives and thereby create new and often pleasurable collective inventions. The return to memory, then, is not a traumatized refusal to live in the present but an active refusal to live in that present *as it is normatively constructed,* a determination to use the past to propose alternatives to current social and sexual systems. The past here offers models for how, if memory serves, the present might be renovated not into a replication of what came before but in the image of the pleasures, intimate arrangements, and social justices imagined by those living now. As Elizabeth Freeman rightly observes, "Sexual dissidents have had to understand what is prior to our own lives with whatever heuristic is at hand: conjecture, fantasy, overreaching, revision, a seemingly myopic focus on ephemera" ("Introduction," 162). Such moments of conjecture and fantasy, cast into the past, make memory central to the work of imagination, drawing forth what Christopher Nealon calls "the 'mythological' features of the texts — their hopefulness, their naïveté" (*Foundlings*, 13). Even as we broaden what Nealon means by "texts" to include television, art installation, street architecture, video, monuments, and film, we want to claim the value of the hopeful and the naïve in relation to memory as a way of imagining other forms of social and sexual life in the face of tendencies to denigrate such imagination as dreamy or impractical.

Such calls on the services of memory are in line with what Michael Snediker calls "queer optimism," a repudiation of "the tropaic gravitation toward negative affect and depersonation" that he notes has "dominated and organized much queer-theoretical discourse" and which he characterizes as "*queer pessimism*" (*Queer Optimism*, 4). Snediker cogently challenges queer theory's "current of enchantment" with negative affects "as sites both of ethics and understanding" (4).[17] We understand the optimism provided by memory in terms of what in chapter 5 we call "ideality," a state that does not foreclose "negative" feelings — one can certainly respond negatively to failures to live up an ideal — but refuses to rest with grief or shame, instead pushing us to imagine more extraordinary versions of the present, generating in the process what, borrowing a phrase from David Eng and David Kazanjian, we call "ideality politics" (*Loss*, 13). By highlighting the difference between that phrase and the now often-discredited "identity politics," which animated earlier discussions of gay and lesbian rights, we mean to signify the movement of ideality beyond (but without necessarily disavowing) identity, allowing for the expansive inclusiveness originally signified by the term "queer." Yet the kinship between these two terms — identity and ideality — suggests as well that the desire for new forms of sociability and community, which animated the optimistic claims made for identity, function similarly as goals for ideality politics. Our hope is that communities founded in ideals rather than (or in addition to) identities might maintain a revisionary social trajectory rather than drifting toward the often inward-directed, essentializing, and therapeutic tendencies that occasionally cluster around identity claims. Ideality is, in short, a politics of the possible, a politics of change and expansion, not a claim to social borders. Idealism has what Carolyn Dinshaw names "a postdisenchanted temporal perspective" ("Theorizing Queer Temporalities," 185) and it is precisely that combination of postdisenchantment and temporal play that makes memory a fitting and potent form of optimistic idealism, providing what Lee Edelman sarcastically calls "the dollop of sweetness afforded by messianic hope" ("Theorizing Queer Temporalities," 195).

Such idealism, derived from the past and oriented toward the present, makes memory serve the vision embodied by every narrative, object, and site examined in the following chapters, whether in the impromptu AIDS memorials and fantasized "homelands" of marked gay spaces of memory; in the chatrooms that testify to the desire of young people, gay and straight, to engage the kinds of cultural literacies circulated on the television sitcom *Will and Grace;* or in novels, films, and videos that depict scenes of remembering as the means to social activism and sexual pleasure. Far from heeding the call to unremember the past and to distance themselves from previous generations, queer artists, filmmakers, novelists, sitcom writers, architects, and memorialists have taken up memory with a vengeance, turning pastness into a potent tool for inventive sexuality, expansive sociality, and creative activism in and for the present. Within these memories, if we remember (the causes and consequences of) amnesia, we might be able to dance again at ground zero.

1. BATTLES OVER THE GAY PAST

De-generation and the Queerness of Memory

De-generation

"All profound changes in consciousness by their very nature bring with them characteristic amnesia," Benedict Anderson claims, explaining the rise of national identity from a deep historical and historiographic dialectic of memory and forgetting. "Out of such oblivions, in specific historical circumstances, spring narratives" (204). In this chapter, our attention is on the forming not of national or supercultural identity, as it is for Anderson, but of subcultural or countercultural identity. In particular, we are interested in calls for gay men to forget the sexual cultures forged by previous generations of gay men. Such calls for what we refer to as de-generational unremembering prescribe amnesia as a prophylaxis against loss. In these calls, loss is the seemingly inevitable inheritance bequeathed by the sex radicals who, because of their careless and adolescent hedonism in the 1960s and 1970s, brought us AIDS. Since the early 1990s, the United States has experienced a profound shift in sexual subjectivity, and as Anderson argues will occur with any deep shift in consciousness, the change has provoked a systematic operation of unremembering. Contra Anderson, we argue that narrative does not follow in the wake of amnesia but precedes it. We do not accept that "amnesia" follows in an inevitable dialectic that produces narrative in its wake but rather that unremembering is the product of narratives that interpellate sexual subjectivity in the image of a historical lacuna or a willed forgetting. The years following the onset of the AIDS epidemic witnessed a discursive operation that instigated a cultural forgetting of the 1960s and 1970s, installing instead a cleaned-up memory that reconstitutes sanctioned identity out of historical violence. Like national identities, the sexual consciousness that emerges from such narratives of forgetting and sanctioned memory serves state interests, not least by turning gays and lesbians into a "respectable" (fit for assimilation) constituency ready to receive state recognition in the form of "rights."

De-generational unremembering was at the heart of the culture of the sex panics — the systematic assault on sexualities that diverge from the interests of the privatized and heteronormative reproductive family — that reached a fever pitch in the United States in the final years of the twentieth century. Sex panics, such as the crackdowns on nonnormative sexual spaces by the police or by zoning boards, are outgrowths of restrictive changes in cultural consciousness.[1] We argue, then, that the assault on gay memory and the resulting modification of sexual consciousness was a necessary precursor to the "urban renewal" projects of the mid- to late 1990s in cities like New York, which in the name of health and touristry (touristry *as* health) closed bars, bathhouses, porn theaters, and other spaces where public sex took place. Acts of memory generate and justify a different sexual consciousness, which in turn shapes divergent theories of the relationships sexual subjects — and here we are talking especially about urban gay men — have to one another and to ideas about social protest and cultural organization.

Consider two stories we received from gay men in response to earlier versions of this chapter, both testimonies to the shifting connections between memory, sexual subjectivity, and activism. The older of the two men wrote:

> I found myself experiencing quite a bit of "Seventies envy" lately — probably not an uncommon experience for gay men under 35 or 40. And it's not really about the unlimited, worry-free, AIDS anxiety-free sex. It's more about the kind of intimacy you can experience in public sex spaces. In fact, my first such experiences shocked me because I was

so surprised how much better I was treated by gay men in those spaces as compared to other gay social spaces. Even rejection is kinder and gentler, and in group scenes, you end up having sex with men who you might not have sex with otherwise — men who are both more and less attractive than you are. Not to idealize it, but it struck me as a relatively democratic and inclusive space as compared to gay bars, for instance (which is not to say that hierarchies don't get enacted — The Unicorn would be much worse than the backroom at the Ram, for instance).

Anyway, when someone stuck poppers under my nose for the first time, I felt like I was actually transported back to the Seventies. I felt like I was feeling what "they" must have felt, our older (or dead) gay brothers (dare I use that term), some of whom were actually in the room, symbolizing the historical continuity that so often gets obscured by discourses of ageism. I felt like I had tapped into some eternal, car-nal, homoerotic AND brotherly stream of consciousness. Essentialist and sentimental, yes. But I experienced a much greater sense of com-munity than, for instance, I ever did in cliquey and self-righteous ACT UP and Queer Nation social circles. And guess what? I started going to demonstrations again (ones that benefit lesbians, too!).

The second man, roughly ten years younger, has a very different story to tell. His narrative begins with his graduation from high school in 1992, but he quickly (in the second sentence) urges us to "fast forward" two years to his recognition in college of his newly formed identity as a mem-ber of Generation Q(ueer).

As a fairly representative member of the elite of "Generation Q"....
I feel fairly safe in saying that activism, per se, is gasping for its final breath before falling into oblivion. The reasons are numerous, and with a small amount of investigation obvious. For decades, centuries even, there was a prevailing feeling of fear and discomfort at the concept of being a gay individual in society. And it simply no longer is an issue for most people who are entering adulthood in the late 1990s. Grow-ing up I, as well as numerous of my friends, were not confronted with the sort of oppressive anti-gay imagery that activism works so fever-ishly to eradicate. We don't feel oppressed, we don't feel limited, we don't WANT to feel the need to be a "united front" — rather what we see is a culture among gay young adults that is far, far more concerned with individual concerns and causes. This was a trend that began years ago, it would seem.

However, in the 1980s what occurred was a regeneration of activist spirit to fight AIDS. Well, it's been years now—and the community understands it. And frankly, among many (though I do not speak for all) Generation Q'ers there is a prevailing feeling that "no one has a body that's good enough to die for." Essentially, the sympathy is no longer there—if someone doesn't practice safe sexual practices, then it is THEIR problem. And what we have is a condition in 1990s America that operates as laudanum for the activist spirit. And you know what? That's not bad—in fact, it should be embraced. . . . It has come to the forefront of young gay intellectuals that by SEPARATING and SEGREGATING themselves from the rest of society they are in essence setting back the clock decades. I feel comfortable in speaking from the perspective of a young gay man who moves in circles of the relatively cosmopolitan. And as such, allow me to address the major difficulty for us in terms of activism, as evinced in the 1970s. It evokes images of the "whore culture." Who would have thought that "gay college guys" and "monogamy" would be used in the same sentence without any negation? Activism had always focused far too much on "embracing" gay culture rather than improving it. . . . Some say that it is a matter of the abrupt and visible tendencies of the under 25 Queer culture to be considerably more conservative than the over 25. Rather, I see it as a subconscious rejection of what we are not comfortable with. . . . People had not been exposed to information that said "yes, you can be gay and have civilized, happy, dating relationships that don't involve casual sex with whatever guy you find attractive.". . . It has finally occurred to Generation Q that to make any significant progress in our own lives (call it greedy, if you like) that it's time for gay men to stop thinking with their dicks (excuse the expression) and start thinking about the future. The Buzzword, so to speak, of Generation Q has been POST GAY. Although rather amorphous in definition, it is essentially this feeling that "queeny protest" is out—and getting on with our lives as productive members of society is in . . . our energies are better spent elsewhere on the question of gay prosperity.

One could draw many conclusions from these two accounts, but we want to focus on the use both men make of memory in sorting out questions of sexual culture, identity, and activism. Both accounts are memory narratives that attempt to orient the reader by offering an experience from the past. Yet the second writer expresses a desire to "fast forward" from the past in order to "start thinking about the future." The first account, in contrast, takes up the consequences of memory only in its final sentences. Not surprisingly, given their different reactions to "dwelling" in the past, the two men arrive at different judgments of a previous generation of gay culture. While the first writer expresses desire, fondness, even "envy" for the 1970s, the second views that decade with distaste. Locating the 1970s as the originating moment of "whore culture" and "queenly protest" (both phrases that reflect, in slightly more crass form, the sentiments espoused by gay neocons throughout the period in which these narratives were written), the second writer invokes memory only to shape it as unhealthy, thereby distancing himself from the past, whereas the first account, full of envious longing, imagines a connection that is in part real (both generations join in the activities of the backroom) and in part fantastic (what the writer calls "sentimental"). The amnesia the second man works toward (he is writing against those who would "turn the clocks back") implies distance not just from the past but from collectivism: now that "the sympathy is gone," there is no longer any need for a "united front" (although in what might be a memory trace he speaks repeatedly for an entire generation). The key terms in the second man's understanding of progress are "comfort" and "prosperity," best accomplished through monogamous coupling and dating, as opposed to "group scenes," of proud and enterprising individuals ("individual concerns and causes"). The chief values expressed in the first account are quite different, relating to a "democratic" and "inclusive" intimacy that is both sexual and collective.

Of course, neither man is completely representative of his generation, although each claims that representative status for himself, speaking in a collective voice. And yet, the attitudes they articulate reflect broader shifts in values around economic and social issues that characterized the last fin de siècle. In their specifics, their accounts remain richly evocative of competing attitudes toward memory and collective action (whether of sex or protest or both) that lie behind recent sex panics and prosex activism in cities such as New York. Our motive is not to assess which of the competing "memories" of the 1970s conjured by these men is empirically more accurate, whether, that is, gay men in the 1970s "actually" experienced anything like sexual democracy or irresponsible abandon. Rather, our interest lies in what the desire for memory or for forgetting allows each writer to inscribe in the *present* in relation to his consciousness as a gay man. For the first writer, memory allows him to generate—for himself if for no one else—a *communitas* that authorizes his activism on behalf of social transformation. In contrast, we worry about the second writer's assumptions—that activism has died and that advances in gay visibility and acceptance are real and permanent—not despite but *because* of the things the second writer sees as most characteristic of his generation. While we commend the second man's confidence that "gay is good" and his dedication to safe sex, we worry that these have been purchased through a kind of brutal each-man-for-himselfism and a restrictive definition of who can figure as the exemplary gay. We argue, further, that the first account, with its faith in collectivism, social expansion, and sexual inventiveness, is more desirable as a narrative of "queer" sexual culture and as an antidote to current restrictive attitudes and policies toward nonnormative sexual practices than is the vision expressed by the spokesman for a generation that claims to be more queer than its predecessors but nevertheless endorses individual prosperity, private coupling, and intellectual comfort, what the writer considers the exemplary values of "civilization."

What we ultimately want to claim is that placing memory in the service of social formation may not leave us locked in an irrevocably lost past but may help us *in the present* to resist normativity (hetero- and homo-) and to enhance erotic and social imagination. Key to that change from willed forgetting to purposeful memory is a shift in emotional registers from shame and guilt to desire and elation. As the historian John Demos long ago noted, guilt is the touchstone in a disciplinary regime that seeks to make the values of the industrializing nation internalized as the freely chosen discipline of individual citizens. Sex panics rest on a pedagogical structure that uses guilt about a past, forgotten and then resurrected as dirty, selfish, and diseased, to instruct subjects in the "proper" values that, as Demos notes, are logically contradictory: on the one hand the expansive opportunity promised by individualism and on the other the regulatory self-control that the individual practices to prevent her- or himself from fully experiencing that potential. We do not claim that the acts of countermemory we are advocating are *not* invested in disciplinary pedagogies. They are. The struggle one sees in the first account, in which the writer seeks to place himself in a cultural setting where he feels he both does and does not belong, demonstrates that this account, too, is a parable of identity-formation and the necessary self-alienations (the condition of "envy") it produces. Yet given a choice between these two technologies of memory and identity, we would still argue that strategic countermemory is crucial to transformative activism in the queer present and future.

Neoconservative gay journalists such as Gabriel Rotello, Michelangelo Signorile, and Andrew Sullivan achieved unprecedented visibility in mainstream media by repudiating attitudes they associated with the generation that preceded them.[2] These men were criticized by Michael Warner for blaming AIDS on gay sexual culture and calling upon New York City authorities to regulate the places where sex occurs.[3] Grievous as these invitations to state regulation were, they were just part and parcel of a larger strategy to vilify queer memory. Justifying governmental crackdowns on queer sex, gay neocons enacted a form of de-generational amnesia, cutting gay men off from memories that provide alternative models of sexual and political community.

In a National Public Radio (NPR) *All Things Considered* segment, "Sex Clubs and Bathhouses Again Popular with Some Gay Men" that aired June 1, 1995, for example, Rotello began his case for closing the baths and sex clubs by drawing a sharp distinction between the unhealthy behaviors of those traumatically rooted in the past and the healthy vision of those who can leave that past behind:

> On the one hand is the specter of governmental involvement in gay sexuality, which is something that I don't think that any gay liberationist or self-respecting gay person welcomes. On the other hand is the specter of a continuing epidemic that will continue to take the lives of 40 or 50 or 60 percent of all gay men. A rational person would have to say that the danger of a permanent epidemic is worse. But, unfortunately, in the gay world, many people, on this particular subject, are not rational. Many people are so traumatized by their past as gay men and by the stigma, and they see the resistance of that as their primary motivation in gay liberation, rather than actually the saving of their own community from this cataclysmic holocaust.

"In the best of all possible worlds," NPR reporter Joe Neel continued, "Gabriel Rotello wants a twenty- to thirty-year period of what he calls sexual conservatism, where gay men have far fewer partners than they do today. That, he says, would break the chain of infection. But that also means a complete break with the past. Gay men must totally rethink the way they conceive their sexual behavior." Rather than focusing on the historical connections between "normalcy" and its constitutive "stigma," Rotello blamed the sexual culture of gay men for the "holocaust" of AIDS. In so doing, Rotello established "sexual conservatism" as the healthy outgrowth of a willed amnesia, the sine qua non of gay public life. In this NPR story addressed to a national audience, Rotello's claim that HIV transmission is the inevitable result of gay men's traumatic attachment to a pathological past enhanced the segment's paternalism, dressing disciplinary normativity in the drag of liberal benevolence.

Taking its cue from Rotello, the segment became a normalizing exercise in the restructuring of gay male memory. In one case, Mike, a "thirty-something professional" HIV-positive gay man, recounted an experience in a New York bathhouse. Telling Neel, "I became, first, kind of surprised at the amount of chances I had to infect other men," Mike remembered an experience with a younger man who was willing to have unprotected sex until Mike revealed his seropositive status, at which point the younger man tensed up and left. "I spoke to him later," Mike told Neel, "and he said, 'I'm really angry that I was ready to take that chance.'" From Mike's anecdote Neel concluded, "In this atmosphere of uninhibited male sexuality, men forget about safe sex." But another lesson could have been derived from Mike's story: that one of the two men *didn't* forget about safe sex. Not only did a gay man take responsibility for a stranger's health, the later conversation between the two men demonstrates the communication networks that can arise from "anonymous" public sex, making the circulation of information and compassion possible. Despite the evidence provided by Mike's anecdote, however, the NPR reporter attached a normative moral to a gay man's memory, a dynamic that becomes even more obvious when the reporter moved on to gay historian Allan Bérubé, who told a dissenting story about "uninhibited" gay sex:

> For me, it's the adventure of meeting someone you don't know and feeling this erotic charge and, you know, exploring them and their bodies

and having conversations and having this kind of bond with someone that you never met before and may never meet again. There's this
specialness about this kind of intimacy with a stranger, that there's
nothing else like it and it's its own thing. . . . There can be magic in
those moments that really have a lot to do with trusting strangers. And
there are very few places in this society where that can happen.

Neel again glossed this gay man's testimony to produce a conventional
moral. Despite Bérubé's description of the trust that can arise in "anonymous" sex, an account seconded by Mike's bathhouse memory, Neel declared, "In New York, closing some places did send a message to the
gay community that danger lurked in bathhouses and clubs." Here trust
established among gay men through sex cultural codes and presented in
the form of a memory narrative turned into a tale of lurking danger. Gay
voices were credited in this nationalized account only when, like Rotello,
they denounced the hedonistic trauma of the gay past and not when, like
Mike or Bérubé, they attested to alternative public intimacies authorized
by gay countermemory.

Attempts to authorize sexual conservatism by normalizing gay memory rely on a strategy we call "de-generation," a look back in fury that
represents the sexual "excesses" of the pre-AIDS generation as immature,
pathological, and diseased, and that diagnoses willed forgetting as prophylactic health. Such arguments for unremembering operate within a
wider discursive assertion that death necessarily marked a gay man's future
because sin characterized his past. This blame game makes illness proof
positive that the afflicted have lurked in the dark dens of perversion, relin-
quishing all claims to compassion, comprehension, or credibility. Under
pressure from AIDS activists and critics who challenged this narrative of
blame, the story shifted from individual "victims" to the practices of sexual culture more generally, a supposedly less cruel because more abstract
gesture. Even if individual gay men were not genetically or psychologi-
cally programmed for self-destruction, this story goes, the culture these
men produced, centered on reckless perversion and unthinking abandon, contained the seeds of death and dissolution. A morbid and pathologizing essentialism is thus displaced from individuals to the collective.

The danger of such de-generational unremembering is not only that
it represents the past inaccurately but that it limits options for nonnormative identification, intimacy, and pleasure. The recent resurgence

of assimilative political initiatives—for gay marriage and military service, most notably—are sustained by narratives that, in the guise of exposing a corrupt sexual past, directly or implicitly urge queers to distance themselves from the tainted past and to structure their lives along cleaner, healthier lines that end up replicating normative heterosexuality. Working in a culture of sexual paranoia so profound that such ideological work is easily carried out in the guise of "common sense," de-generational unremembering represents sex as a fixed object of moral evaluation, obscures the dominant culture's role in establishing sexual "norms" as a technology of power, and denies the agency of "deviants" who use unsanctioned sex to challenge the normalizing structures of mainstream America.[4]

Sexual De-generation

De-generational assertions were not the exclusive province of obvious neocons like Rotello. Similar assertions in cultural and theoretical productions of "queerness" throughout the late 1980s and early 1990s anticipated the pervasive deployment of de-generational unremembering by gay neocons in the late 1990s, and thereby unintentionally contributed to the restrictive conservatism of contemporary sexual culture. Some of these texts are surprising. Leo Bersani's influential 1987 essay "Is the Rectum a Grave?," and Gregg Araki's much heralded 1992 film *The Living End* might at first seem as far from Rotello as queers can get from neocons.[5] In retrospect, however, both exemplify a de-generational unremembering that makes queerness compatible with mainstream social values.

In "Is the Rectum a Grave?" Bersani casts the "extraordinary opportunity" generated by the most "malignant" "responses to AIDS" (198) as a "salutary" opportunity to undo the "illusory" fictions generated in "the late 60s and 70s" that gays might come to be perceived as a community within American culture (204) and the related depictions of sex as community-building. The unremembering of gay sexual culture here is performed as the articulation of a set of facts gays always knew: "all gay men know," he says, that "if you're out to make someone you turn off the camp" (208); "anyone who has ever spent one night in a gay bathhouse knows" that it is "telling a few lies" to claim, as Dennis Altman does, a link between that culture and "a sort of Whitmanesque democracy" (206); and, the "big secret" that is revealed in the opening lines, "most people don't like sex" (197–98). Thus the medical and social trauma of AIDS ("Is the Rectum a Grave?" begins as a review of Simon Watney's *Policing Desire*, a powerful condemnation of government and news-media responses to AIDS) is processed as a denial that anything we ever had—community, camp, camaraderie, sex itself—was what we thought we had. In place of these fictions, we are given the truth of the supposedly "ineradicable aspects" of sex as "anticommunal, antiegalitarian, antinurturing, anti-loving" (215). Bersani insists that sex is really a social "dysfunction" that "brings people together only to plunge them into a self-shattering and so-lipsistic *jouissance*" that drives them apart. In particular, the rectum, with its potential for ongoing pleasure and its refusal of the finitude of climax, is for Bersani "the grave in which the masculine ideal . . . of proud sub-jectivity is buried" (222). Welcoming stimuli that shatter ego and hence contradicting "the sacrosanct value of selfhood" (222), the rectum chal-lenges the status of power itself, since, Bersani argues, an ego-affirming sexuality generates a phallic social order. Our concern here is less with Bersani's faith in the devastating psychic power of the rectum (although it fails to account for how an asshole can get fucked and still be an ass-hole) than with how his representation of the relationship between the sexual and the social enables his dismissal of the sociosexual narratives of the 1970s. The ego-shattering potential of the rectum was obscured, according to Bersani, by the "redemptive project" to "rewrite sex" (221) undertaken by such diverse critics and historians as Simon Watney, Jef-frey Weeks, and Pat Califia. These writers, Bersani complains, carried on "the rhetoric of sexual liberation in the '60s and '70s" (219) that, in mak-ing sex the basis of community, identity, or politics, inscribed a phallic logic that disguised sex as "self-swelling, as psychic tumescence" (218). According to Bersani, only Catharine MacKinnon and Andrea Dworkin joined him in having "the courage to be explicit about the profound *moral repulsion* with sex that inspires the entire project" (215). Exposing the deluded sons and daughters of the sexual revolution, Bersani is ready to offer his bottom line: we must acknowledge and celebrate the valuable "humiliation of the self" (217) implicit in all penetrative sex, but espe-cially in the anal sex that is here conflated with gay sex.

While Bersani's de-generational dismissal of the redemptive histories of the 1970s was meant at least in part as a queering of identity (politics), it also positions first women and then gay men within normative sex/gender constructions. In accounting for misogyny, for instance, Bersani claims, "If, for example, we assume that the oppression of women disguises a fearful male response to the seductiveness of an image of sexual powerlessness, then the most brutal machismo is really part of a domesticating, even sanitizing project" (221). But what marked women as "powerless" *prior to* the invention of "brutal machismo"? Bersani answers—and his case for the shattering power of the rectum rests upon this assertion—that women are socially powerless by virtue of being penetrated, passively, by the penis. This formulation begs the question of how sex comes to be known as "penetration" and not, say, "incorporation," a semantic shift that would make the insertee "active" and the inserter "passive." Or what about women who penetrate sexual partners by virtue of prostheses? Or men who can't get it up? Or, on the most basic level, men whose experience of penetration is different?[6] Bersani's assertion of the rectum's power for ego-dissolution thus relies paradoxically on inscribing normative gender in ways that render the sexual subject in the kinds of fixed and limited terms we have no hesitation identifying as essentialist.[7] Bersani seems particularly comfortable generalizing about sex between men who, if one believes the essay, have only anal sex, have never enjoyed sex not centered on the phallus, and lust only after butch tops. The interpellative force of Bersani's essay is clear in his assertions of the "facts" of gayness—the pronoun shift from "all" to "you," for instance, when "all gay men know... you turn off the camp" (208) to pick up men—and is policed on the border of disclosure and duplicity: because "all gay men know" the exclusive desirability of butchness, any gay man who claims otherwise is complicit in keeping a "secret" that only Bersani is brave enough to speak.

Having disavowed other historical accounts of gay male pleasure, Bersani re-creates "real" gay sex in the image of its most conservative straight counterpart.[8] Bersani compares gay "bottoms" in anal intercourse to women who, he joins Dworkin in asserting, can never be "active" during sex. Bersani accounts for violence against children with AIDS, for example, by claiming that they evoke "the infinitely more seductive and intolerable image of a grown man, legs high in the air, unable to refuse the suicidal ecstasy of being a woman" (212). The "top" in both vaginal and anal intercourse, being "phallic," is implicitly masculine, since women, according to Bersani and Dworkin, can never wield the phallus (or, apparently, the dildo).

Bersani's normative rendering of gay male sex as the straight missionary position (no wonder he can claim that the "big secret" about sex is that "most people don't like it") is connected to his assertion that his "rewriting of sex" was undertaken not in response to a decade of antisex rhetoric generated by AIDS hysteria, antiporn feminism, and garden-variety homophobia but because of the widely felt "moral repulsion" concerning the sexual narratives spawned by the late 1960s and 1970s.[9] In Bersani's account, not only does the historical moment of the essay itself get off the hook, its gender norms and anticommunal pursuit of radical individualism are naturalized as essential psychic truths willfully ignored by the writers of the sexual utopianism of the 1970s.

The difficulty of representing alternatives to sexual conservatism once gay men divorce themselves from memory becomes evident in Gregg Araki's 1992 film *The Living End*, in which two gay men, Luke and Jon, respond defiantly to their seropositivity by taking to the road, driving aimlessly, shooting up ATMs, and fucking with and without condoms, in public and in private. The appropriated "road trip" narrative calls attention to and frustrates the abjection audiences had come to expect as an appropriate closure to the story of AIDS, but while *The Living End* refuses to make individual gay men's sexual acts the cause of their inevitable despair and demise, it struggles with a causal narrative of blame (a narrative with which, we believe, it ultimately disagrees). Jon and Luke are caught in a tension between two historical narratives: one that Bersani might call "redemptive" and the other de-generational. Unable to reconcile these narratives, the film's ending is, at best, ambivalent, even desperate. With his characters representing at different moments both sides in the debates over memory, Araki shows they can be brought together as a single unit only with the price of violence and desperation.

De-generation enters the film in the scene following Luke and Jon's first night together, as Luke explains his AIDS-inspired philosophy over breakfast: "So figure this: There's thousands, maybe millions of us walking around with this thing inside of us, this time-bomb making our futures finite. Suddenly I realize: we got nothing to lose. We can say, 'Fuck work.

Fuck the system. Fuck everything.' Don't you get it? We're totally free. We can do whatever the fuck we want to do." Luke's conception of freedom teeters, in this scene, between an oppositional stand toward obligatory capitalism ("Fuck work. Fuck the system") and the hopeless lack of commitment ("Fuck everything") that is, according to conventional AIDS narratives, the teleological necessity of a positive HIV diagnosis. Luke's inability to sustain opposition without lapsing into despair—his "Fuck everything" ends in his later exasperated claim, "I don't care about anything anymore"—appears to arise from his attempt to purchase his "freedom" through generational blame. Immediately preceding the lines just quoted, Luke tells Jon:

> I mean, we're both gonna die. Maybe in ten years, maybe next week. But it's not like I want to live forever and get old and fat and die in this ugly, stupid world anyway. I mean, we're victims of the sexual revolution. The generation before us had all the fun, and we get to pick up the tab. Anyone who got fucked before safe sex *is* fucked. I think it's all part of the neo-Nazi, Republican final solution. Germ warfare, you know? Genocide.

If Luke refuses the closure of despair, if he knows he is not to blame for his own infection, he can claim his innocence only by displacing guilt from the individual to the cultural past. It remains unclear, in Luke's account, how the "fun" had by a previous generation of gay men *and* Republican genocide can both be responsible for AIDS, but both somehow are; the "sexual revolution," rather than constituting a challenge to conservatism, acts in tandem with the political climate that allowed the epidemic to flourish.

Luke's de-generational narrative generates contradictions that come dramatically to the surface at the film's conclusion: while Luke may have wanted to distance himself from a previous generation of gay men whose "fun" has gotten him in his present fix, only by engaging in what Bersani calls the "reinvention of sex" as defiance and as the basis of countercultural companionship can Luke express his anger and achieve the agency that helps him escape isolation and despair. In the film's concluding scene, when Jon, sick and disgusted with Luke's antics, decides to go home, Luke rapes him, holding the barrel of a revolver in his own mouth and vowing to pull the trigger as he climaxes. Just as the film seems to reach the despair that AIDS narratives seemingly required as closure, however, this conventional AIDS narrative diverges at the last moment, when Luke throws aside his gun and Jon, who had slapped Luke and walked away, returns. The film's last shot shows Luke and Jon sitting side by side in the middle of an arid landscape, leaning on one another's shoulder. Once Luke, whose initial speech represented the core of the neocon argument against memory, refuses to hold a gun to Jon's head (a suggestive metaphor), both recognize that each is the other's support, literally and figuratively, in a narrative that, while it does not say where these men might go next, refuses to sentence them to isolation and death-figured-as-suicide.

The film's conclusion implies, then, that Jon and Luke owe more than one debt (the debt of infectious fun) to the previous generation's enabling fantasy of sex-as-community and of sexuality-as-resistance. While degenerational discourses that vilify politics or companionship based on sexual pleasure place Jon and Luke in the overdetermined narratives of inevitable illness ("Anyone who got fucked before safe sex *is* fucked") and despair ("I mean, we're gonna die"), the connections they forge from their sexual pleasures, neither entirely arbitrary, sentimentally idealized, nor ineffective in opposing hatred, prove the most effective tools for resisting the victimizing narratives of heteronormative national culture. Granted, those older sexual narratives could not be resurrected uncritically to meet the political demands of the film's historical moment. Not only had AIDS made it difficult to see some forms of sexual pleasure as liberating (the film associates Luke's desire to be fucked without a condom with his other despair-induced suicidal behaviors), it had rendered problematic the equation of sex and liberty. But this was not because, as Bersani claimed, sex is "anticommunal" or "antinurturing" but because devastating losses despite heroic efforts made liberty itself seem like an impossibly utopian project. If the sexual narratives of the 1970s could not be sustained uncritically, however, neither, the film seems to suggest, should they be left behind. Given the tension between de-generational forgetting and sexually redemptive memory, the film shows the latter, while not perfect, to be its protagonists' best bet for ensuring a living end.

Sexual culture, as Araki's road film makes clear, was never a settled space (when one tearoom closed, the action generally shifted to another), but the memory of practices, signs, and identifications enabled tearooms, discos, cruising areas to travel without disrupting—or at least not for very long—their functions. The impermanence of these spaces, if any-thing, suggests the resilience of the networks through which sexual cul-ture circulates, for, as Berlant and Warner acknowledge, it is relationships that create the queer world. As we have suggested, those relationships are formed through the medium of memory. Crackdowns on space alone could not destroy a public culture predicated, in many ways, upon regu-lation and migration. But a crackdown on memory is another story. We offer these examples of de-generational narratives to show how pervasive the attack on collective and individual memory has been and how closely allied that assault was with the interpellation of gay men within normative public culture. These attacks—as well as the counterattacks represented by films like *The Living End*—conditioned queer culture throughout the early 1990s. Although drawn from three very different genres addressing potentially variant audiences, these accounts reveal how de-generational narratives circulate between subculture (Araki's film) and superculture (NPR), from accounts under attack by queer theory (Rotello's) to the theorists that queers have used to challenge those accounts (Bersani). Demonstrating the false purity of differentiations between theory and journalism, subcultures and national cultures, the circulation of de-generational narratives links these texts in contests over the relationships between and meanings of representation, memory, and identity, struggles that would preoccupy queer culture and politics for the next decade.

Queer Countermemories

Against calls for de-generational unremembering, other narratives that began to emerge in the mid-1990s represent what Foucault called "counter-memory": competing narratives of the past composed from memories that exceed official public history ("Nietzsche, Genealogy, History"). Foucault privileged an ideal of the oral transmission of history over the homogen-izing memories presented in the mass culture of the mid-1970s, which he analyzed in relation to how French identity was constructed in the mass media in ways that denied memories of "popular struggle" ("Film and Popular Memory"). But today, when ever more accessible technolo-gies have provoked an explosion in varieties of mass media at the same time that interpersonal transmission of cultural memories of struggle are stymied by insistent disciplines of unremembering, film, videos, and even television have become an increasingly important means for archiving and transmitting the cultural past. Such changes in technology should alter our assessments of mass culture, even as we remain true to Foucault's fundamental presumption that "if one controls people's memory, one controls their dynamism. And one also controls their experience, their knowledge of previous struggles" (92). In the aftermath of AIDS, when praise of an earlier generation was hard to claim publicly, knowledge of previous struggles emerged in mass media as a specifically queer countermemory, a way to remember the oppositional and creatively sexual gay culture of Foucault's own lifetime, which some of his other essays explored. "Homosexuality is an historic occasion to re-open effective and relational virtualities," Foucault observed, "not so much through intrinsic qualities of the homosexual, but due to the biases against the position he occupies" ("Friendship as a Way of Life," 207). Among the "virtualities" Foucault pointed to are the social relationships developed in the urban queer spaces: "A way of life can be shared among individuals of different age, status, and social activity. It can yield intense relations not resembling those that are institutionalized. It seems to me that a way of life can yield a culture and an ethics" (207). For Foucault, gay desire is itself a form of memory: "For a homosexual, the best moment of love is likely to be when the lover leaves in the taxi. It is when the act is over and the boy is gone that one begins to dream about the warmth of his body, the quality of his smile, the tone of his voice. This is why the great homosexual writers of our culture (Cocteau, Genet, Burroughs) can write so elegantly about the sexual act itself, because the homosexual imagination is for the most part concerned with reminiscing" ("Sexual Choice, Sexual Act," 224).[10] Viewed through the lens of queer memory, intimacy becomes a shared history as much as a shared space. Internalized as behavior patterns through its integration into memorial narratives of pleasure, intimacy becomes the basis for a transformative and erotic collective life.

Gay countermemory has provided oppositional representations of memory's centrality to pleasure that inscribe alternative public intimacies. Contemporary with the trends toward de-generation in the mainstreams of the news media and elsewhere, a variety of writers and filmmakers registered a determination to engage with the past. The ironic titles of three novels—Brad Gooch's *The Golden Age of Promiscuity* (1996), Ethan Mordden's *How Long Has This Been Going On?* (1995), and Felice Picano's *Like People in History* (1995)—suggest the exclusion of gay men and lesbians from conventional history. A mysterious "this" that the mainstream doesn't know is "going on," gay public life, denied a historical "golden age," has existed as what Gooch calls an "intense subtext" (16) of sexual subculture ("promiscuity"). At the same time that they exposed the exclusion of gays from conventional history, these novels deployed countermemories to create communal subjectivity, making sexual culture a site of creative reimagining rather than a dangerous lure or a paradise lost.

In Mordden's ambitious *How Long Has This Been Going On?*, for instance, memory becomes the means to codify and circulate everyday practices, providing gay men with ways to recognize and communicate with each other in the face of violence, death, or dislocation. Mordden renders the relationship of memory, self-invention, and public intimacy most explicit in the story of Jim and Henry, former college classmates surprised to find each other in a New York gay bar. Rather than sharing conventional reminiscences, Mordden writes, "This time they are going to work out a very different kind of nostalgia—whom they had crushes on in college, who else *was*, what exactly they themselves knew they were—the conversation, in short, that marks the two men's passing from acquaintances to comrades" (233). These collaborative acts of self-inventive memory predicated on desire create bonds—"One hour of such talk and you can be intimates for life" (233)—that survive homophobic isolation and the debilitating grief caused by AIDS. When, at the novel's conclusion, Henry, contemplating the present status of gay cultural politics, laments that "probably no political movement in history counted as little solidarity as this one," an act of memory restores his faith. As the Gay Pride march stops to honor the memories of those who have died, Henry remembers his college friend Jim, who died from AIDS the previous year. It's an anguishing moment for Henry, but it also renews his optimism, for despite the lack of solidarity in gay life, "on this afternoon, the feeling was unity. This was the one day when everyone In the Life seemed part of a great striding giant of a history that would never cease its advance" (564).

Mordden's narrative suggests, however, that gay cultural politics were threatened at least as much by the paralyzing de-generational rupture — represented in the novel, as in Bersani, as perfectly consistent with queer "world making" — as by AIDS itself. When Blue, a 1970s hustler turned 1990s AIDS activist, joins a group of twenty-something queers in a chic Lower East Side coffeehouse, he's shocked to hear one woman declare, "Well, *I'm* sick of Old Gay... Drag, and opera, and Fire Island. *Gyms!*" (568). In contrast, the hope for the future, the novel suggests, lies with those of the younger generation who can draw survival lessons from the past. In a scene set during Gay Pride Weekend, 1991, two young lesbians watch a documentary on pre-Stonewall gay life. When one woman asks, "Do you relate to any of this?" her lover responds, "It's not us. . . . But it's something. It's history." "Maybe it'll make sense later on," the first woman ventures, to which her lover asserts, "It makes sense to me now" (559). Only when history "makes sense" — when memory serves — can gay countermemories heal the antagonism generated not by AIDS but by de-generational discourses that make memory-based community a suspect concept.

In a more comic vein, *How Long Has This Been Going On?* shows how memories circulate codes of identity ("what exactly they themselves knew they were"), taking on an explicitly historiographic function predicated on the sex so often hidden from history in the official archives. In the novel, Larken Young tells Frank Hubbard, a Los Angeles vice squad decoy attempting to come out, stories of his sexual past that over time lead Frank to resign from the police force in order to enter the "gay scene." Dissatisfied with remaining in the margins of history, however, Frank decides to take an active role in recording his experiences, transforming himself from vice cop to gay pornographer. Pornography, in Frank's handling, not only conjoins memory with an explicitly sexual content, it also transforms popular memory into an expandable public site of collective sexual pleasure and interpretive recollection. Unhappy with porn's implausible and generic plots, bearing no relation to gay life as he knows it, Frank decides to write and star in his own films, which quickly become gay classics. In his first film, a "pleasant-looking but unerotic young man" arrives on Fire Island, knowing no one. Eventually he has sex with a series of men and, after each encounter, takes on some aspect of his partner's apparel, until he is ultimately transformed into a sexy leatherman.

At the end of the film, through trick photography, the newly created leather-hero fails to recognize his former self when they pass one another on the beach. Frank's film tells a somewhat unconventional coming-out story, but one that proves recognizable to those in the audience who, like Frank, have learned how to survive and prosper as gay men not through official channels of instruction — religion, family, education — but through encounters, often sexual, with other men: his memory narrative becomes theirs. As one audience member responds, "I am in this film" (400).

Because Frank's film self-consciously debunks conceptions of memory as a transparent relation of an "actual" past (remember the trick photography) and presents "identity" not as something given but as something learned in experience's postmortem, its memory narrative resembles Freud's theory of melancholia. For Freud, the melancholic, refusing to relinquish his or her libidinal attachment to a lost object, incorporates aspects of that person into him- or herself. Mordden's novel offers a witty account of how sexual subculture may serve as the lost "object" of queer melancholy, having been "lost" in the sense both that individual lovers have moved on and that the culture as a whole has disappeared in the face of AIDS and de-generational unremembering. Refusing to forget, Frank's protagonist becomes not self-lacerating in the ways Freud described melancholics as becoming but more determinedly fierce and self-possessed as a result of his psychic preservation. In this regard, Mordden's novel seems to echo Douglas Crimp's powerful 1989 essay, "Mourning and Militancy," which argued that gay men's refusal to "lose" friends and lovers to AIDS had given rise to the bold militancy evident in activist groups such as ACT UP (*Melancholia and Moralism*, 129–50). Neither mourning nor memory is a sign of loss, for Mordden or Crimp, but of erotic literacy, subcultural belonging, and living commemoration in the face of real and symbolic death. Frank's porn is not only his history; it is the record of his melancholy transformation into gay historiographer. Frank's porn films offered an enabling representation of memory and community for their gay male viewers not because they were viewed as transparent representations of an essential "gay life" or of the historical period they purport to represent but because they provided inventive opportunities to engage memory as an imaginative act of *generation*, creating narratives that reflect and revise a hybrid combination of "the

codes, the terminology, the system" and "behavioral styles" of the remembered past and the remembering present.

For Freud, the subject refuses to "lose" his or her libidinal object because of residual ambivalences toward that object. Melancholia is not a
simple celebration of the past, therefore, but contains elements of critical
correction as well. Seen in this way, gay countermemories may be as critical
of the kinds of representations generated by Mordden as they are inventive in imagining divergent queer codes and styles, as one sees in Gooch's
The Golden Age of Promiscuity. Watching gay culture evolve through the
1970s from a frenzy of self-invention in the emerging culture of New
York sex clubs and leather bars to a predictable performance of standard-
ized deviance, one character worries that "gay life might wind up being a
snore" (94). Gooch's narrator, Sean Devlin, "felt aroused by freedom. But
freedom and identity were canceling each other out" (42). To avoid being
"canceled out," Sean, who always felt gay life to be "a surface of images"
(35), becomes, like Frank, a maker of films that revise his personal experiences into representations of communal reinvention. Rendering the gay
bar scene as representation, Sean reintroduces the interpretive flux for
which gay men's sexual culture, according to Gooch, is especially suited.
Far from bringing the end of shared endeavor, rendering gay memory as
an interpretable — and variable — text makes it once again a site of communal self-invention as well as of prescription. Describing the cast of his
film, Sean says, "By now a lot of the men from the Shaft had shown up
in the movie.... If they were a tribe, they were an improvisatory tribe
with no set tests" (203–4). For Gooch, as for Mordden, the formation of
improvisatory tribes becomes possible through the circulation of sexual
memory narratives that constitute a "snippet of history" (300), while such
provisional formations in turn constitute a "golden age" of gay public life.

The various and often divergent depictions in these texts of what constituted gay life in the 1970s — S/M clubs and piano bars, disco divas and
gym clones, porn and police raids — makes abundantly clear that no one
narrative of gay urban culture in the 1970s will represent the "real" story.
Memory is not transparent, a simple reflection of what actually "was."
Gay countermemories will often differ and sometimes collide. Nevertheless, the acts of renovation explored in these texts lead to, in Foucault's
words, "the appropriation of a vocabulary turned against those who had

once used it" ("Nietzsche, Genealogy, History," 154). Gay countermemory becomes self-defense as it intervenes in de-generational unremembering, engaging the gay cultural past—particularly the sexual cultures of the 1970s—to challenge imperatives toward irrevocable loss, isolating individualism, generational division, and social conservatism. To look back is, after all, to refuse the imperatives laid down at the destruction of Sodom. In these countermemories, the "sexual revolution," rather than causing AIDS, offers codes of intimacy and the models of communal preservation that contrast the abstemious and individuating ways of life developed in the eighties. That gay countermemories emerge in these novels through the figure of filmmaking is indicative of the way parts of the mass media became a site of resistant queer memory.

One of the first instances of mass media enacting queer memory was the 1990 film *Longtime Companion*. The fact that it was heralded as the first cinematic treatment of AIDS pitched at mainstream audiences predisposed activists to be critical, and some in the crowd booed the director and author when they spoke at a New York Gay Pride rally in 1990. David Román has analyzed in some detail the attacks on *Longtime Companion,* noting that critiques of its focus on a community of white gay men were repeatedly voiced by "white activists and critics perhaps uncomfortable with their own viewing" (293). We would analyze this discomfort as part of the traumatized will to forget that characterized gay and queer culture by 1990. The film re-creates with startling accuracy the look of the 1980s and, more poignantly, in Willy's (Campbell Scott) baffled failure to say or do the right thing in the face of overwhelming devastation, some of the emotions of that decade that are most painful to recall.[11] Reflecting an understandable—perhaps strategically useful and psychically necessary—preference for militancy over mourning, hostile critics singled out the film's final scene, which depicts the three surviving characters (including Willy) walking on the beach at Fire Island, imagining the moment when a cure is found for AIDS. Suddenly, crowds of cheering people, including the characters who have died, come running onto the beach, embracing their living friends. Attacks on this conclusion as a manipulative and sentimental suggestion that losses to AIDS could be recovered, even in fantasy, were countered at the time by Simon Watney, who put forward an appreciative reading of the film's ending as a representation of "the most simple and passionate wish that none of this had ever happened, that our dearest friends might indeed come back to life again, that we miss them horribly. This is surely not to be dismissed as 'denial' or 'delusion,' but should be understood as a necessary catharsis, and moreover a catharsis that binds our communities even closer in their fight to save lives" ("Short-Term Companions," 163).

Returning to this scene now, what is striking is how specifically it addresses the relationship of community and memory. This accords with what Román rightly notes as "among the film's most significant achievements" overall: "its insistence on presenting AIDS as a collective social experience" ("Remembering AIDS," 296).[12] The scene on the beach in 1989 is preceded by one set in 1988 at a cabaret benefit for people "Living with AIDS," a powerful phrase eventually coined by activists to counter mainstream characterizations of "AIDS victims." An actor, Howard (Patrick Cassidy), whose transition from closeted careerist to activist has been one of the plots the film follows, now introduces himself as "living with AIDS." He then introduces a trio of musicians who perform the Village People's 1978 hit "YMCA" set as a ballad accompanied by cello, clarinet, and guitar. This performance of a song now associated with the time just before AIDS seems at first to provoke confusion in the audience, which turns to glee when it becomes clear that it is intended as a fond satire. This demonstration of the power of memory—reworked for a new context—segues through the guitar soundtrack to nine months later when, it is implied, Howard has died and just three of the film's original characters have survived. Returning to the Fire Island beach where the film began, we see that we are in a symbolic landscape: in contrast to the bustling crowds of scantily clad men who populate Fire Island at the film's start, the beach is now deserted and bleak, although we are told it is July. The conversation is presented in one continuous shot, emphasizing the continuity that binds this trio of friends. Beginning with a discussion of their commitment to an upcoming ACT UP demonstration where they plan to be arrested, the talk turns to the crisis of memory caused by AIDS. "It seems inconceivable, doesn't it, that there was ever a time before all this," Willy asks. In response, his companions turn to the blame narratives about "sleeping around" that characterized so many responses to AIDS. "It's just not the point," responds Willy, "I'm sick of hearing people pontificate about it." He then shifts to trying to imagine the future:

WILLY: I just want to be there if they ever do find a cure.

FUZZY: Can you imagine what it'd be like?

LISA: Like the end of World War II.

This invocation of collective, cathartic relief drawn from history provokes the fantasy of everyone who has been lost to AIDS returning, the hordes of people streaming down the boardwalk to repopulate the beach with their joyful reunions, depicted against a soundtrack of Zane Campbell's "Post-Mortem Bar," in which the singer narrates having "cleaned out your room" and "painted the walls to cover any memories." Despite this effort to suppress memories, however, the singer nevertheless feels like his dead friend is "hovering over" and "keeping an eye on" him. The song's repeated refrain runs:

> And we'll go down to the post-mortem bar
> And catch up on the years that have passed between us
> And we'll tell our stories
> Do you remember when the world was just like a carnival opening up?

The song is a prescient description of the battle over gay memory at the start of the 1990s. Despite efforts to "cover any memories," those memories still hover protectively. The losses represented by the pastness of memory cannot be recovered, for years "have passed between us." But that very pastness allows gay men to "tell our stories" as an act of invention as well as remembrance, combining the elements of fantasy and recollection that comprise the reunion scene on the beach. As Campbell sings these lyrics again, the fantasy disappears, the beach is once again deserted, and Willy reiterates his wish: "I just want to be there." The referent of "there" now is ambiguous, however: "there" is not a spatial location but a time that incorporates both the future after a cure, the past when all these people were joyously living, and the present represented as a fierce determination to survive, individually and collectively (the "there" in this sense refers to an upcoming ACT UP demonstration the three characters have just been discussing). The power of this scene lies not in a naïve belief that the losses due to AIDS can ever be magically recouped but in a more complicated fantasy not of recovery but of continuity. The fantasy is of gay men — and the woman who represents the importance of their allies in the queer community — using their memories of the past to strengthen their bonds with one another and their determination to fight with and for one another, with the help of their memories, in the present and future.

While novels such as *How Long Has This Been Going On?* and *The Golden Age of Promiscuity* and films like *Longtime Companion* suggest the importance of countermemory for sustaining the cultural practices of gay men who came of age in the 1960s and 1970s (even as they remember those practices differently), and who have experienced the decimation of their social networks by AIDS, a number of video makers focused on the value of countermemory for younger queers coming of age in a post-AIDS era. Their videos assert, contra de-generational imperatives, that the past is an invaluable tool for generating intimacy and for strengthening resistance to the isolation, guilt, and despair caused by unremembering. In Raoul O'Connell's 1995 *A Friend of Dorothy,* the protagonist, Winston, sets off to Greenwich Village to begin his freshman year at NYU armed with his Barbra Streisand, Bette Midler, and Cher albums. These singers, whom a homophobic character in the video identifies as "fag divas," provide Winston with comfort and, ultimately, a boyfriend. While shopping for a Streisand CD, Winston makes eye contact with a man perusing the Judy Garland selections. After camping for a few moments, the boy asks Winston if he is "a friend of Dorothy's," pre-Stonewall code for "Are you gay?" When Winston answers, "Yes, I guess I am," the man responds, "Someone should teach you to smile when you say that," and asks him out to, of all nostalgic locales, a piano bar. The video ends by suggesting that icons and codes of the gay cultural past continue to provide places to meet, signs of identification, and modes of communication necessary to self-esteem and collaborative pleasure.

Robert Lee King's 1994 *The Disco Years* took viewers back to the disco fever of 1978 when Tom Peters, a straight-acting, straight-appearing high school athlete, begins to realize his homosexuality following a one-night stand with a fellow athlete, Matt. Trying to reassert his heterosexuality, Matt joins a group of students in terrorizing a gay teacher, writing homophobic epithets, and taping male centerfolds on his classroom walls. When Tom identifies the vandals to school authorities, an anonymous caller notifies his mother that her son is gay, and Tom, fleeing his mother's tears and "it's just a phase" philosophizing, ends up at the local gay disco where, as Tom's voice-over makes clear, he could "be around people who would accept me the way I was." The final scene of the video underlines the message that seems to structure *A Friend of Dorothy* as well: the gay cultural past offers young gay men the vocabulary through which to imagine, if not absolute freedom, then liberty from the individuating, lethalizing subjectivities provided by de-generational accounts. As the soundtrack plays Cheryl Lynn's "Got to Be Real" and the film shows Tom disco-dancing with the high school's much vilified queer, Tom's voice-over, itself a marker both of memory and historical distance, explains, "In time the world of gay dance clubs would prove to be a trap of its own. But for now none of that mattered. At last I had found a place where the dance floor was filled with people like me. And the air was charged with a sense of freedom and excitement. And disco." Without negating the passage of time that would make "the age of disco" a "trap" and its recovery impossible, King's video performs memory as a means of survival useful in the present ("for now") precisely because its pastness gives fantasy (whose small town ever had such a disco?) the aura of authenticity and suggests, by so doing, the possibility of materializing similar fantasies in the present.

The creative possibilities enabled in the present by the fantasized reconstructions of the past become the direct content of Mark Christopher's 1994 *The Dead Boys' Club*, which, without denying the irretrievability of the past, makes that irretrievability and the resultant fantasy behind any memory into an opportunity for invention and pleasure. In the opening sequence, the mise-en-scène suggests that the young protagonist, Toby, is torn between two generations: in one hand he holds that depressing AIDS emblem, a bottle of bleach, which he brings to his cousin who is cleaning up following the death of a friend; in the other he holds one of the best-known accounts of the gay male sexual revolution, Andrew Holleran's *Dancer from the Dance*. The impact of that novel becomes clear when Toby cruises a man on the street and takes his phone number, but the antiseptic and antisex ethos of his own day reasserts itself, and Toby throws the number away. Yet the vision enabled by Holleran's novel doesn't simply disappear: rather, it is translated into the campy camaraderie of Toby's cousin and his friends and, more pressingly, as the fantasy content that underlies Toby's own experiences of memory.

In the following scene, the viewer is introduced to Toby's gay older cousin, Packard, and Packard's friend Charles, a swishing, wig-wearing queen of the old school who immediately begins to hit on Toby. The video's contrast between the anxious and undersexed young man and the humorous, sociable older men highlights the generational change that is its central concern and shows that cultural values of the past become more, not less, valuable in the context of AIDS. When the video introduces the older gay men, they are packing up the belongings of a friend who has just died from AIDS. Their wit and shared memories comfort them in grief. For them, AIDS is not the denouement in a narrative of selfish recklessness but the decimation of a gay culture essential to survival, especially for those caught in de-generational imperatives. When Toby doesn't know who disco diva Donna Summer is, Charles laments, "Your generation will never know what it missed," to which Packard responds, "I think they do."

The video's principal trope highlights the contrast between the sexual austerity of the present and the sexual inventiveness of the past. Packard gives Toby his friend's favorite "slut shoes," and when Toby tries them on, he is given a miraculous view into the "sexual underworld" of the 1970s, placing him among scantily clad men in leather cruising dark, disco-filled corridors. Freaked out by his transmission into the past, Toby at first tries to throw away the shoes, but, representatives of the repressed cultural unconscious that they are, they continually return to him. When he wears them out to a bar one night, he gets picked up by the man whose phone number he threw away earlier on the street, and when he wakes up in the morning in this man's bed and finds the condom Packard gave him still unopened in his pocket, Toby assumes, in the logic of de-generation, that his glimpse into the older sexual culture has led him to reckless, unsafe sex. The past has risked his health, Toby believes, and he refuses to see his one-night stand when he returns the shoes Toby left behind. The film draws the reader away from Toby's de-generational conclusions, however, showing us the open condom packages under the bed that Toby cannot see. One-night stands, bar culture, disco — none of these is antithetical to responsibility and health, the video suggests. On the contrary, like Mike's story in the NPR segment with which this chapter began, old-fashioned sex culture can become a site not only for companionship and pleasure but for the exercise of responsibility and protection as well.

The Dead Boys' Club acknowledges that we cannot return to the past, for AIDS has changed that past as much for Packard and Charles as for

Toby. But to disavow the past, to deny its representational importance for the present, is equally futile, as the trope of the continually returning shoes demonstrates. The past will not be left behind; like the protagonist of Gloria Gaynor's disco hit, it will survive. And if Toby wants to survive as a sexually active gay man, he must accept the past, embracing the sense of erotic and pleasurable community organized by the previous generation around the shared signifier "gay," an older sexual culture that developed the ethos of "safe sex." Realizing this, Toby finally reconciles the present with the past in the video's final scene: the last time Toby throws the shoes away, a street merchant finds them and places them among his wares. When Toby, rethinking his rejection, reaches for the shoes, his hand touches that of another young gay man, who is also reaching for them, and they smile at one another as the video ends. This scene is the allegorical center of the video: two gay men are brought together pleasurably by their common reach for the past, by memory. We don't know if either man buys the shoes, and that doesn't matter. Returning to the past *in fact* is less important that the collective act of reconstructing that past, by the desire for *pastness,* that constitutes memory. While completely reentering the past is an impossibility (signified by the contemporary production of 1970s footage rather than using footage filmed *in* the 1970s), the "past" will not be left behind (the closing credits run over Thelma Houston's disco hit, "Don't Leave Me This Way") but will be rendered as cultural discourse, as countermemories, that enable new and more pleasurable narratives today: endings-in-sex rather than the sex-as-ending that de-generation prescribes.

We conclude with a film that self-consciously combines the elements of memory, invention, mediation, and political survival after AIDS that this chapter explores. Gus Van Sant's 2008 *Milk* returns to events in the emerging gay rights movement in San Francisco, culminating in Harvey Milk's 1977 election to the San Francisco Board of Supervisors and his assassination by another supervisor, Dan White, the following year. The film avoids being either a faux documentary or a transparent historical re-creation by repeatedly citing an earlier documentary, Rob Epstein's powerful 1984 *The Times of Harvey Milk.* Over the course of *Milk,* Van Sant repeatedly quotes Epstein's film by returning to the archive to retrieve film clips used in the earlier documentary, by re-creating scenes from Epstein's film, and by taking footage directly from *The Times of Harvey Milk.* These scenes challenge the deployment of unmediated news coverage often presented as reliable "fact" on television or in documentaries. Above all, these scenes suggest the recycled nature of memory itself: viewers who were present in San Francisco might remember the events depicted, as would viewers of Epstein's documentary. Memory thus appears not as an individual or unique possession but as a process of citation and re-creation invoked to serve the needs of the present. Memory, the self-conscious citations of *Milk* suggest, is collective and mass mediated, collective *because* mass mediated. The effect of visually quoting a documentary that was itself a shaped construction of gay countermemory (Epstein's documentary was released in the year of Ronald Reagan's reelection, a political victory for the antigay advocates of "family values") allows memory to affirm relationships among sexuality, inventiveness, and political daring even while acknowledging that such an importation from the past is a projection backward from the present. The relay from 2008 to 1984 to 1978 also suggests the continual, if latent, presence of pastness, of recollection, in the cultural imaginations of gay men across the apparent temporal watershed of AIDS. Generating what might be called metamemories, twice- (or even thrice-) told tales that point explicitly to the intertextuality rather than the transparency of memory, *Milk* marks a second-wave metamemory of post-AIDS countermemories, a recollection of previous recollections of a time before AIDS.

To claim *Milk* as a metamemory is not, it should be clear by now, to accuse it of derivativeness or inauthenticity. On the contrary, by combining mass media, memory, and self-conscious citation, *Milk* approximates more closely than Epstein's earlier, more straightforwardly archival documentary the structure of Harvey Milk's political efficacy. At every dramatic juncture of the film, Milk tells his friends and staff to assemble a crowd and to call the media. Having created these audiences, Milk performs for them moments of poignant memory, most famously recalling the phone calls he receives from young people around the country who speak of their desperation and express their gratitude for the kind of activism taking place in San Francisco. These anecdotes are pitched to evoke in Milk's gay and lesbian auditors memories of their own childhoods, an implication that becomes explicit in *Milk* when he challenges the young and not yet politicized Cleve Jones with, "What was it like to be a little queer in Phoenix? Did all the jocks beat you up in gym class?" It is not necessary that memories be ideal or sentimental, the film suggests;

they can be of painful experiences as well (memories of childhood persecution or, in the context of the film, of Milk's assassination). What *does* matter is the collectivizing capacity of memory despite its content. The citation of memory in Milk's stump speech, its translation into mass media (both news coverage then and film re-creation now) even as it was used to swell emotion in a present crowd, demonstrates the efficacy of memory narratives—even traumatic ones—in building political community when they are consciously invoked and turned into collective reparative action. This emphasis on collectivity is contrasted in *Milk* with the anti-identitarian assimilationist strategy of more mainstream gay politicians and media executives, represented in the film by David Goodstein, owner of *The Advocate,* and Rick Stokes, who ran against Milk for supervisor. Goodstein tells Milk he'll never win public office until he abandons his counterculture identifications, stating, "You're too old to be a hippie, Harvey Milk!" This assimilationist conception of progressive time, moving individually and politically from infantile self-indulgence to mature self-restraint, each stage of development replacing and eradicating the previous one, is countered by the back-and-forth temporal movements of the film, which compress past and present in ways that undo sequential order (the variety of temporal frames in Milk's rhetoric is emphasized by the plural "times" of Epstein's title). Milk refuses to surrender his identifications in the name of a collective political population ("I'm not the candidate," he tells Goodstein and Stokes in the film, "the movement is the candidate") made possible by memories carried through media to other gays and lesbians who can absorb them as their own. In contrast, when Goodstein recounts his own story of antigay discrimination, the lesson he draws from it is that it is safer to be discreet and to appeal to established authorities for accommodation. Significantly, two of the scenes recycled from Epstein's video involve footage of the crowds at San Francisco's Gay Pride celebration and of the candlelight march after Milk's assassination. The recycling of memory throughout a community constitutes that community as a political entity, comprised along the lines of gay identity that, in Milk's articulation, includes a sense of allegiance he phrases as an expansive sense of "us": "it's about the 'us'es out there," Milk states, "not just the gays, but the blacks, the Asians, the seniors, the disabled—the 'us'es." Media and memory, identity and coalition, citation and sentiment: these were not oppositions for Milk, as they have become in so much queer criticism of his "times" today. In the late 1970s, these ideals worked in tandem to generate the political hopes that made Milk's election possible.

Memories serve the needs of the present, as well as of the past, and *Milk* subtly locates its contemporary need in the yoking of AIDS and memory. *Milk* situates the crisis of memory in the context of AIDS by making Cleve Jones, who was consultant on the film, the most prominent character in the film after Milk. Jones, as viewers familiar with the history of AIDS know, founded the NAMES Project, the massive quilt commemorating those who died from AIDS, and another example of how memory inspires gay activism that quickly expanded into coalitions with other constituencies (as discussed in chapter 5). It is not enough to "remember" AIDS, the film suggests; those who remember must understand the connection of post- and pre-AIDS life, of Cleve Jones *and* Harvey Milk, not to blame the latter for the former but to show how the rituals and rhetoric of memory developed in the 1970s enabled the activist response to the epidemic, just as Milk mentors Jones into his life as an activist. Materializing these connections, *Milk* turns the memories in the film into memory *as* the film, generating a mass-media countermemory of gay political and collective hope pitched to resist the current climate of unremembering. It is worth noting that the one sequence of *The Times of Harvey Milk* that Van Sant does not incorporate is the White Night riots that end the earlier film. The riot that followed Milk's assassination becomes, in this way, memory's unfinished business, the missing piece for viewers who "remember" either the history or Epstein's documentary. That missing piece in the film may also be the piece that is often missing in today's queer world: outraged remembering and the coalitional, idealistic collectivity it enables.

While not as self-conscious as *Milk* or *The Dead Boys' Club,* all of the countermemories addressed here, by virtue of their status as art rather than history, refuse a notion of transparent memory, that what viewers see in these films, videos, and novels represent what gay men experienced *in* the 1970s. What the "sexual revolution" meant to gay men then—as various and contested as that was—could never be what it means now. The memories people share are diverse and divergent, and tensions among memory narratives are a necessary part of the continual evolution of gay culture(s). An important reminder of such productive tensions is provided by one of the most eloquent memory narratives on film: Marlon Riggs's 1989 *Tongues Untied*. In his powerful documentary of the often violent tensions between African American and gay cultures, Riggs describes life in 1970s San Francisco with an eye to its (and his own internalized) racism:

> I pretended not to notice the absence of black images in this new gay life, in bookstores, poster shops, film festivals, even my own fantasies. Something in Oz was amiss, but I tried not to notice. I was intent on my search for my reflection, love, affirmation, in eyes of blue, gray, green. Searching, I discovered something I didn't expect, something decades of determined assimilation cannot blind me to. In this great, gay Mecca, I was an invisible man. I had no shadow, no substance, no place, no history, no reflection.

Tied to Riggs's condemnation of gay male racism ("I quit the Castro, no longer my home, my Mecca"), however, is a certain longing, a sense that a more inclusive Castro *would* have been a Mecca, or at any rate a refuge from the homophobia Riggs also condemns in the African American community. Riggs engages in a double act of memory — looking back at the Castro but also back at African American history and his personal home life — in order to create from the doubled rememberings a hybrid memory narrative that allows him to tell his story. Riggs's soundtrack mixes black gay divas (such as Sylvester) with Billie Holliday and Nina Simone as it mixes footage of the March on Selma with that of Gay Men of African Descent marching in a Gay Pride parade. From these mixings, Riggs diversifies gay memory ("Each gay community does different things," one man in the documentary says, "and I think that's cute") and allows a remembering that works for black gay men ("older, stronger rhythms resonate within me, sustain my spirit, silence the clock"). Far from replicating *the* values of a historical moment, Riggs's countermemory corrects the shortcomings of those values and enables new representational possibilities for the creation of a more viable multiracial gay community. By "silencing the clock," refusing a progressive notion of time, Riggs is able to imagine what was useful in the past while amending that past for the present.

In looking at these examples of queer countermemory, we want to underscore the important role memory plays in the making and breaking of queer worlds. By taking too casual an approach to memory, we risk letting our historiography disastrously change our history. The politics of memory are particularly important in relation to AIDS. Even before the NAMES Project made memory into a stirring art form, a common refrain in the gay community was that we must not forget those who have died. While these individual acts of memory are urgently important, we must also remember and continue to shape and deploy our memories of social networks, political strategies, and cultural theories, not to idealize or to reinvent the past but in order to think critically about what stories are credited with access to the social "real." Only in so doing will gay men's sexual representations transform the restrictive and normalizing cultural trends of the 1990s that grew from de-generational unrembering, allowing us to avoid unnecessary loss and become present to ourselves.

2. FOR TIME IMMEMORIAL
Marking Time in the Built Environment

To Mark or Not to Mark

Between 1984 and 1992—that is, while fear and grief over AIDS, the previous chapter argued, played out in proscriptions against queer memory—the French historian Pierre Nora was supervising a massive (seven-volume) study of what he influentially termed *lieux de mémoire,* places of memory. These memory sites, which include both physical places and rituals of commemoration, Nora contends, characterize modernity. Places of memory, Nora argued, enact self-conscious efforts "to block the work of forgetting" that is inherent to the "acceleration of history" in "our hopelessly forgetful modern societies, propelled by change" ("Between Memory and History," 7, 19, 8). We take his influential phrase, generated as part of a study on the spaces of French memory, as the starting point for this chapter in order to emphasize two points: that the assaults on gay memory described in chapter 1 took place at a time when sanctioned forms of memory were thriving and that these campaigns of memory-making were often focused on physical locales.

Minority sexual identities have a long history of withstanding forms of critique and scrutiny not visited upon sanctioned forms of identity—

like heterosexuality or Frenchness—that, in theory, should offer equally valid fields in which to debate biological causality, perform linguistic deconstruction, or outline the sequences of contingent historical events that got us where we are. Spaces of gay and lesbian memory may emerge the stronger for the intellectual rigor to which they have been subjected. It is hard to imagine any critically viable theory of sexuality that would allow for the fuzziness of Nora's defense of memory sites founded on a contingent "will to remember" ("If we were to abandon this criterion, we would quickly drift into admitting virtually everything as worthy of remembrance," he says [19]) but nevertheless justified by an appeal to a lost "real memory—social and unviolated" (8). Nor should theoretically informed critics leave unchallenged Nora's claims that there once were authentic "*milieux de mémoire,* real environments of memory," assertions grounded in romantic notions of "peasant culture, that quintessential repository of collective memory" where "real memory" was "retained as the secret of so-called primitive or archaic societies" (7–8).[1]

While we are not eager to import into queer theory the muddled reality claims in this highly respected theorization of history organized around national identity, we want to use Nora—and the fact of his influence on more mainstream identity constructions—to critique the complete denial, within much queer theory, of the significance of memory-places to identity. For many theorists of sexuality and the built environment, "queer space" is insistently cast in the present. "There Is No *Queer Space,* Only Different Points of View" was the title of Brian McGrath's installation for the 1994 *Queer Space* exhibition at the Store Front for Art and Architecture in New York. This statement ran at eye level along a semicircular Plexiglas screen showing computer-generated images of various Manhattan locales. The project statement explained, "'Queer space' exists potentially everywhere in the public realm . . . it is the individual's appropriation of the public realm through personal, ever-changing points of view." Echoing this claim, historian George Chauncey opened a 1996 article subtitled "Gay Uses of the Streets" with the assertion, "There is no queer space; there are only spaces used by queers or put to queer use" ("Privacy Could Only Be Had," 224). The restriction of queer space to definitions premised on action or perception in the present was reiterated in the 1997 anthology *Queers in Space,* where the architect-turned-artist Jean-Ulrick Désert insisted, "A queer space is an activated zone made proprietary by the occupant or *flâneur*" (21).

Similar claims have been made at the scale of the single building. In 1994, as part of the Wexner Center's *House Rules* exhibition, architects Benjamin Gianni and Scott Weir presented "Queers in (Single-Family) Space," a design for a suburban house configured on the inside to accommodate a variety of living arrangements. Gianni and Weir tied their design's flexibility to the looseness of the term "queer" but rejected any further links. "Sexuality exceeds the purview of the architect," they said; queerness "is more a strategy than a space" (Gianni et al., "Queerying (Single Family) Space," 57).[2] Whether in the landscape or at home, these arguments run, queerness is constituted not in space but in the body of the queer: in his or her inhabitation, in his or her gaze. When he or she goes away, according to this logic, the queerness disappears, leaving none of the traces that might constitute a place of memory.

In 1997, the design historian Aaron Betsky opened his provocative book *Queer Space* with an evocation of the Manhattan dance/sex club Studio 54 in the 1980s, which he posited a paradigm of "queer space" precisely because it was outside time. About "the spaces that appeared and disappeared there every night" thanks to the wizardry of lights and props, Betsky says, "Exactly because they did not stick around long enough to accrue meanings, memories, or emotions, they confronted you much more clearly as nothing but pure space, activated only by your own body" (5). Transcending time, this version of queer space rejects claims to both the past and the future. "Inside Studio 54," Betsky asserts, "a new world was born, but it would have no issue, it would make no difference, it would save nothing. It was pure act" (4). Memory plays no role in this ideal of Studio 54 as a paradigm of queer space. Even the queer space of collectors who acquire and display historical artifacts Betsky characterizes as a product of fantasies in the present — "building up a fantastical world by gathering objects from all times and places" (10) — rather than engaging a relationship to the past.

But can it really be that we leave no traces and have no relationship to the physical embodiments — the places and things — of the past? More to the point, should such amnesia be our theoretical ideal for queer space? On the contrary, we argue that queerness carries with it a particularly important relationship to places and things. As Sara Ahmed reminds us, the concept of "sexual orientation" is based on a spatial metaphor: "If we know where we are when we turn this way or that way, then we are orientated. . . . To be orientated is also to be turned toward certain objects, those that help us to find our way" (*Queer Phenomenology,* 1). And despite theoretical imperatives to unremember, there have been fledgling efforts at defining the spaces of queer memory, mainly maps and walking tours to identify and publicize spaces associated with the history of queer communities (Dubrow, "Blazing Trails," 281–300; Martinac, *The Queerest Places*). A vast array of texts about the queer past—from personal memoirs to histories of places like Cherry Grove, New York City, and Philadelphia—attest to a broad desire to ground sexual identity in history.[3]

Even Betsky's *Queer Space* is driven by a yearning for memory. It begins as a memory narrative—"Looking back on it [Studio 54], this was a queer space" (5)—and deploys a rhetoric of defiance against forces of modernization very similar to those Nora articulated in relation to a disappearing "peasant culture" as the raison d'être for *lieux de mémoire.* "AIDS destroyed the queer community as a coherent structure, and queers disappeared into their homes, the suburbs, and anonymity," Betsky says, adding, "They adopt children, dress like their neighbors, and even disavow the presence of a communal culture" with the result that "queer space is, in fact, in danger of disappearing" (192). Betsky also shares with Nora a focus on the role of place in creating identity. Queer space, Betsky says, "has shown all of us how to create identities that depend on real experiences and connections with other humans to create a community" (193). Despite its stated indifference to memory, Betsky's book is cast against a normativizing amnesia, becoming itself a queer *texte de mémoire,* a self-conscious construction of the past arranged to counter memory losses that would impoverish the present and the future. The monuments and markings discussed in this chapter speak eloquently to a similar desire to leave traces: to create environments that engage the history of minority sexual identity, to cherish and to use the memories they provoke.

Pride and Prejudice: The Monuments

The increased visibility of sexual identities in the 1970s gave rise to a concomitant desire for visibility in the form of public monuments. These

spaces of memory were pedagogical as well as commemorative, asserting the presence of same-sex relationships for a heterosexual public and
consolidating identities in relation to history for gay and lesbian viewers. What remain to this day the two most prominent *lieux de mémoire*
associated with sexual orientation—the *Gay Liberation* monument in
New York and the *Homomonument* in Amsterdam—were both commissioned in 1979. Queer theory's antipathy to the historicity of space has
guaranteed itself (tautologically) through a conspicuous critical neglect
of these spaces. Even the *Gay Liberation* monument at a busy intersec-
tion in Manhattan's Greenwich Village—arguably the most visible public marker of gay identity in America—has attracted almost no scholarly
attention.[4] Its fraught history, which resulted in a thirteen-year lag between its commission in 1979 and its installation in 1992, offers a remarkable register of changing attitudes toward both sexual identity and
art during this tumultuous period. It's a great story, with a cast including an earnest activist (Bruce Voeller, the first executive director of the
National Gay Rights Task Force) and an eccentric philanthropist (Peter
Putnam, a multimillionaire who worked as a night watchman and janitor
in Houma, Louisiana).[5] Several carnivalesque public hearings featured
spokesmen for the Catholic church warning that children would be corrupted by the sculpture, as well as neighborhood groups competing to
display lists of signatures on petitions ("Now *that's* show business," one
witness commented when a pro-sculpture group encircled the entire meeting room with a ribbon of pink petitions containing almost thirty-five
hundred signatures [Saslow, "A Sculpture," 24]). The four models for the
figures showed up in t-shirts with the motto "Grotesque Stereotype" in
response to attacks on the piece (Boyce, "The Making of *Gay Liberation*," 12). Homophobic opposition was matched—in rhetoric, if not in
numbers—by complaints that the monument, indeed that any artwork,
was not radical enough. "We believe that legal and social equality for gay
people is the only proper monument for the heroic Stonewall Rebellion,"
announced the Gay Activists Alliance (Saslow, "A Sculpture," 26).

This history of the sculpture also reflects the dynamics of the art world,
where, clichés of avant-garde radicalism notwithstanding, the donor's insistence on a well-known artist collided with the fact that artists generally
get famous by claiming a "universal" relevance inimical to overt identification with historically subordinated identities.[6] Initially, the sculptor

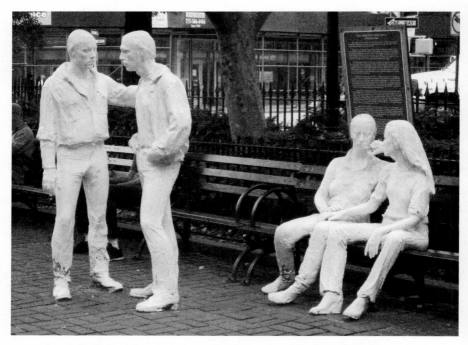

George Segal, *Gay Liberation,* Greenwich Village, New York, white bronze and park benches. Commissioned 1979; dedicated 1992. Photograph by Christopher Reed, 2009.

Louise Nevelson accepted the commission, "remarking almost gleefully that she had grown too old and too famous for anyone to hurt her at this stage in her career," but she was persuaded by her "business advisors" that acknowledging her lesbianism would hurt the career of her younger lover, and she pulled out (Saslow, "A Sculpture," 27).[7] None of the other prominent, but closeted, artists approached by the funders was willing to be identified with a project about homosexuality. The commission, there-fore, went to George Segal, an uncontrovertibly heterosexual artist fresh from a controversy over his Kent State memorial (funded by the same benefactor), whose commitment to the project fit comfortably with the avant-garde's history of addressing (speaking about), rather than being identified with (speaking for), social marginalization.

It's hard to fault Segal's goodwill. He turned his signature style — life-size white body-casts of real people — to a commission that specified that the work "had to be loving and caring, and show the affection that is the hallmark of gay people. . . . And it had to have equal representation of men and women" (Saslow, "A Sculpture," 27). Explaining his decision to accept the commission, Segal said, "I'm extremely sympathetic to the problems that gay people have. They're human beings first. I couldn't refuse to do it" (in Summers, "George Segal's *Gay Liberation*"). Segal created two casts of the work, one for New York and the other for Los Angeles. When the California cast was severely damaged by vandals after its installation on the Stanford University campus, Segal said, "It shocks people to express the opinion that a homosexual is a decent, sensitive human being — and I'm shocked at that" (in Saslow, "A Sculpture," 28).

Good intentions aside, however, it can't really be said that *Gay Libera-tion* ever filled the need Voeller articulated when he explained that "on his nationwide travels for NGRTF. . . one of the questions he most fre-quently encountered was, 'Why are there no memorials to Stonewall?'" (in Saslow, 26). The peaceful figures, denounced by activists as "all white, thirtyish, and middle class," hardly evoke the riot between police and the Stonewall Inn's regulars, as recalled by Thomas Lanigan-Schmidt: "STREET RATS, Puerto Rican, Black, Northern and Southern whites, 'Debbie the Dyke,' and a Chinese queen named 'JADE EAST.'" Nor, despite the late-1970s hairstyles apparent on close observation, does the sculpture of two tentatively touching couples do much to recall that moment of sexual ex-perimentation and (often) gendered essentialism that characterized the time it was commissioned, let alone the in-your-face AIDS and queer activism of the 1980s and early 1990s, during which the piece was end-lessly debated and delayed before finally being installed in 1992. Indeed, the couples' apparent indifference to each other or anyone else (art crit-ics called it "deadeningly somber" [Saslow, "A Sculpture," 28] and com-plained that the "figures seem to have withdrawn . . . into a rigid, autistic blankness" [Kimmelman, "Sculpture, Sculpture Everywhere"]) suggests that if *Gay Liberation* monumentalizes any moment of sexual identity, it may be the dystopic vision of couple-centric anonymity Betsky decries as the millennial collapse of "queer community." Although it stands at a — ar-guably *the* — significant site in queer history, the banality of the figures in *Gay Liberation* contributes to its failure to create a place of memory. The integration of the life-size figures into the normal activities of the park manifests a laudable ambition to distinguish this modern monu-ment from the conventions of, for instance, the nearby statue of General

Sheridan on his high granite plinth. But as James Saslow said of the figures when they were exhibited in a Manhattan gallery in 1981, "They are too mundane, too paltry an image to radiate even a fraction of the beauty, wisdom, and excitement which 'the special brand of affection that is the hallmark of gay people' has come to mean to me" ("A Sculpture," 31).

More alert to the distinctive bonds Saslow associates with sexual identity is another monument, which was also commissioned in 1979, although this one was completed in 1987: the *Homomonument* in Amsterdam. "Naar Vriendschap Zulk een Mateloos Verlangen" ("For friendship such an unmeasurable longing") is the inscription on the *Homomonument*, which sits in the Westermarkt, a picturesque open area between a canal and the back of a seventeenth-century church.[8] The designer, Karin Daan, chose this line from a poem by Jacob Israël de Haan partly for its connections to the history of Amsterdam (de Haan's most famous poem, quoted on a memorial to him near the Rembrandt house, concerns the nostalgia he feels shuttling between his home cities of Amsterdam and Jerusalem). About "For friendship such an unmeasurable longing," Daan explains:

> This sentence is so beautiful because it's going straight into the heart, it is intense and unlimited/immense (mateloos) and has a special meaning for homosexuals because of the Dutch connotation in the word VRIENDSCHAP (friendship) with Homo Love: "de liefde die vriendschap heet": "the love which is named friendship." It is also the title of a book of homoerotic poetry by Hans Hafkamp [published in] 1979. I decided this was the best sentence to create a bigger time and space. It's a very open text, it has its meaning for everyone in his own way, it's clear and beautiful. It's as the homomonument is, an open space where life is going through.[9]

As Daan's explanation suggests, the *Homomonument* engages issues of history and sexual identity in an open-ended way that is also manifested in its disposition as three elements in the urban fabric. Unlike the Segal (or other more traditional sculptures), the *Homomonument* does not demand attention for itself as a symbolic object but instead charges the physical space of the city with meanings born of memory. Composed of three massive pink granite triangles recalling the labels the Nazis used to persecute homosexuals (the way Jews were marked with yellow stars),

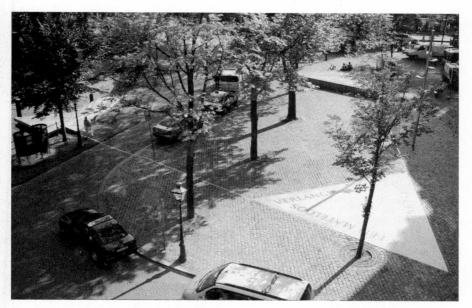

Karin Daan, *Homomonument,* Westermarkt, Amsterdam, pink granite. Commissioned 1979; dedicated 1987. Photograph courtesy of Karin Daan.

the *Homomonument* is not shy about alluding to a history of gay oppression.[10] Memory here is not conceived in opposition to performativity in the present, however, for the placement of the elements at some distance from each other—one flush with the cobblestone pavement, one stepping down into the canal, the third raised like a dais—integrates the monument into the flow of daily life. Necessarily perceived in fragments, the *Homomonument* creates a space not immediately noticeable but then suddenly overwhelming in its scale, propelling viewers into active awareness of their participation in a zone that is both spatial and temporal.

The history of the *Homomonument*'s commission and design reflects this emphasis on collectivity. Drafted by a committee representing the gay/lesbian subgroups of several political organizations, the call for designs described a "'living' monument" that, in addition to commemorating a history of oppression, would become a site for the exchange of "information about current events in the struggle for gay liberation" and "serve as a centre for demonstrations" (Koenders, *Het Homomonument,* 28).[11] The jury that selected Daan's design praised the way "the symbolic character of the pink triangle and the various elements of the memorial, protest and pride, spill over into the city" (42). Fund-raising was carried out throughout the Netherlands. Today, the success of the *Homomonument* may be gauged from its popularity as a site of queer pilgrimage, marked with daily floral tributes and annual ceremonies of remembrance and celebration.

Engagement with memory was central to the conception and commission of the *Homomonument*. The ad soliciting proposals listed three criteria (aside from an ability to withstand vandalism):

- The Homomonument must commemorate gay men and women who in the past were persecuted and oppressed.
- It must also be a sign that the current gay liberation movement is active in the struggle against rape, discrimination, and oppression. It must show that as a gay man, woman, boy, or girl you are not alone.
- It must be a call for permanent vigilance, it must challenge the accepted role patterns of man and woman. (Koenders, *Het Homomonument*, 38)

The pink triangle motif evokes both the Nazis' use of the symbol in the past (a reference intensified by its proximity to the Anne Frank memorial) and its reappropriation as a badge of pride by gay men and lesbians at the time the monument was created. In selecting Daan's design, the jury praised the way one point of the triangle gestures toward the Frank house and another toward the headquarters of a nearby gay/lesbian center.[12] These historical allusions have been central to the reception of the *Homomonument*. Literature issued by the organization responsible for the monument notes that the gay/lesbian center is "the world's oldest continuously operating gay and lesbian organisation" and describes the third point of the triangle (the one stepping down into the canal) as pointing toward Dam Square at the heart of Amsterdam, where gay activists were arrested in 1970 for attempting to lay on the National War Memorial a lavender wreath commemorating the homosexuals killed by the Nazis. The *Homomonument*'s historical references are explained in a flyer, which draws attention to the temporal dimension of the monument, interpreting the three triangles as "symbolizing the past, present, and future. . . . A war memorial that only recalls a past laid in stone would ultimately be worthless. A monument must be equally grounded in the present and look to the future."[13]

The differences between these two monuments are instructive. *Gay Liberation*, while located at a historically significant site, forecloses connections between the events it supposedly commemorates and the styles, personal and artistic, of its own moment, much less between those moments and any future viewing moment in which observers might want to imagine new identities through reflections on the past. The *Homomonument*, on the other hand, engages pastness as an opportunity for current creativity, collectivity, and action on the part of sexual minorities. The past, these monuments both show, cannot be abandoned if the history of sexual resistance and innovation is to continue into the present and future. But neither can memory be, as it were, set in stone: it must remain open to interpretation, adaptation, and innovation, allowing people in the present to connect creatively with those who came before. That is how static monuments become Nora's *lieux de mémoire*, places that marshal narratives of the past in order to form and strengthen resolve, pleasure, and courage in the present and future.

Imminent Domain: Places

In order to invite participation in the present, monuments might avoid the temptations of didacticism in favor of the possibilities of what we have called "imminence," a readiness to take place (Reed, "Imminent Domain"). Apart from the repeated element of the (subtly) pink triangle, none of the historical references associated with the *Homomonument* is explicit to viewers; even the Anne Frank house, although its proximity clearly contributes to the site's meaning, is around a corner, out of sight. The richness of the associations accrues as a sequence of realizations, building incrementally to an overwhelming sense of scale, even while inviting viewers to seize, claim, and create from references to a past not gone but imminent in the present. Designed so that it continually reenacts this dynamic in relation to the bustle of urban life passing through and around it, the *Homomonument* seems related less to other monuments than to more vernacular spaces of queer memory, which exemplify this concept of imminence.

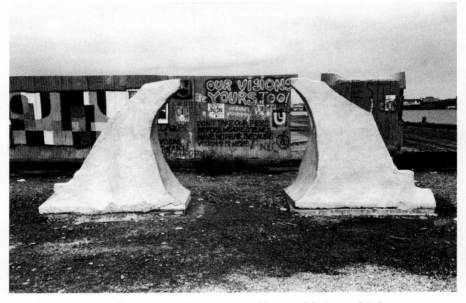

West Side piers off Lower Manhattan, 1970s–80s. Photograph by Leonard Fink.
Courtesy of the Lesbian, Gay, Bisexual, and Transgender Community Center
National History Archive.

As with other forms of public life in contemporary America, however,
queer claims on space are tenuous. Many vernacular sites of queer memory have been lost. The most famous of these disappeared environments
is probably the abandoned commercial piers along the Hudson River off
Greenwich Village in Manhattan. A site for sunbathing and sex as well as
a gathering place — and sometimes a temporary home — associated with
gay teenagers, transvestites, and transsexuals, the piers became a locus of
memory, marked by casual graffiti — much of it, as the AIDS crisis developed, explicitly memorial — and elaborate decorations, most notably the
vast sexual tableaus — "paintings of mythical sexual figures — devils in
sunshades fucking tattooed, muscular satyrs" (Sember, "In the Shadow,"
219) — by the artist who called himself Tava.[14] All these disappeared when
the area was turned into a park in the 1990s.

A similar now-disappeared environment was the Rocks along the shore
of Lake Michigan in Chicago's Lincoln Park near the so-called Boys Town
neighborhood. Here a revetment of massive limestone blocks stepped

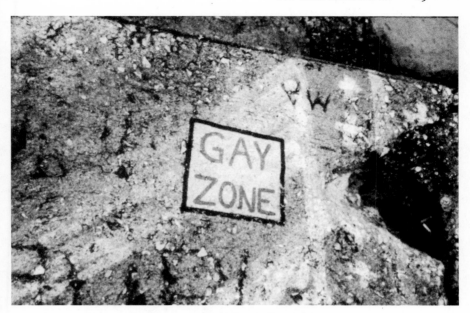

Revetment, Lincoln Park, Chicago. Photograph by Christopher Reed, 1995.

down from the grassy park into the lake, providing a sheltered area for sunbathing and cruising. As on the piers, graffiti executed with various levels of care marked this stretch of revetment as what one vignette called a "Gay Zone." The Rocks were symbolic enough of the neighborhood to give their name to *Off the Rocks*, a Chicago journal of gay/lesbian creative writing founded in 1981. As on the piers in New York, the graffiti assumed an increasingly memorial aspect as the AIDS crisis wore on. Red ribbons were painted on the rocks and decorated the carefully tended little gardens that began to intrude from the top of the revetment onto the hard-packed grass of the park at the water's edge. Like the piers, this space has also disappeared. Despite community efforts to preserve the painted stones, they were lost between 2003 and 2006 when the revetment was rebuilt in a way that precludes secluded sunbathing (or whatever else goes on in seclusion). Today the Rocks are recorded primarily in works of art. In 2002, a German artist, Alexander von Agoston, created a mural-scale (ten by ten feet) painting of the Rocks as a preemptive memorial to this threatened space—painted on both sides, the canvas depicted a group of men on the Rocks in swimming suits and towels on

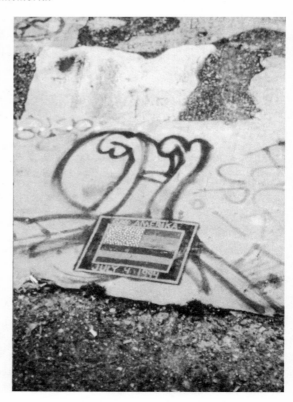

Revetment, Lincoln
Park, Chicago.
Photograph by
Christopher Reed,
1995.

one side and naked on the other (von Agoston, "Belmont"). In 2009, the
photographer Doug Ischar exhibited a series of photographs of the Rocks
under the title *Marginal Waters*. Ischar presents these images, which were
shot in 1985, as an act of remembering: "Understand that from the get-go
I was photographing gay men almost out of a sense of desperation because of AIDS. I was fearful AIDS would obliterate queer culture. I had
this fervid conservationist mission." Exhibiting them twenty-five years
later, he says, "There's a sad disconnect in gay life between generations.
Young gay men don't know the art my generation made, and they don't
know older gay men. This is like families without grandparents. It really
saddens me. If this work makes even a slight contribution to that, I'll be
very pleased" (Heidemann, "Sonny and Sheer").

Other cities no doubt have manifested such collective and ad hoc interventions into the landscape, though these have gone undocumented.

Interventions by sexual minorities into the vernacular cityscape seem to fall between phenomena that attract scholarly and journalistic notice: forms of performance (from street demonstrations to practices of cruising) associated with queer subcultures on one hand and forms of street-marking (graffiti and murals) associated with ethnic and racial subcultures on the other. Between these much discussed manifestations of urban inhabitation lies a rich culture of spaces marked by sexual minorities, exemplifying neither the dead time of official monuments nor the ephemeral nature of performance, but something both more contingent and more legible than most accounts have acknowledged.

There is, of course, truth to claims that queer culture often circulates through spaces nominally marked for other purposes, from the avenues taken over for demonstrations to the wooded areas, bathrooms, and warehouses taken over at certain times for sex. These exemplify the adaptability of sexual minorities living without sanctioned institutional spaces. Without wanting to deny or devalue the importance, socially and theoretically, of such environments, we challenge the way such "unmarked" spaces (and how unmarked, really, are those often highly scrutinized spaces of public sex such as bathrooms?) get generalized into the totality of "queer space," especially when such claims ignore or denigrate the variety of deliberately marked locations in which gay life takes place.[15] In denying the presence of marks or traces, such generalizations risk erasing the inscription of memory and the adaptations of such memories to contemporary needs that, as Nora theorizes, make cultural collectivity possible.

To idealize what we might call the stealth homosexual, who cruises parks and back alleys undetected, is to valorize an image of the queer as loner or as victim, as in flight from or trapped by a stigmatized identity. A recent memorial in Berlin to those persecuted by the Nazis for homosexuality takes up these ideas of invisibility and hiding, presenting itself on first glace as an anonymous concrete shed that seems to mirror the spaces privileged by queer spatial theory. Viewers may choose to peer through a small window at a short black-and-white film of two young men kissing in a park. Unlike the monuments analyzed in this chapter, this piece, by the Danish artists Michael Elmgreen and Ingar Dragset, was conceived as what James Young influentially called a "counter-monument," a visual rhetoric in which Germany calls "on itself to remember the victims of

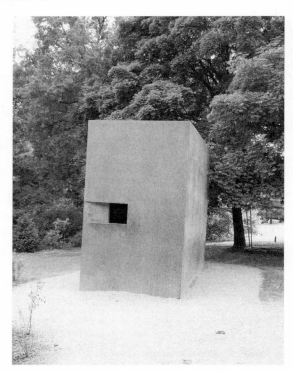

Michael Elmgreen
and Ingar Dragset,
*Memorial to the
Persecuted Homo-
sexuals,* Berlin;
dedicated 2008.
Photograph, 2008.

crimes it has perpetrated" ("The Counter-Monument," 52). Young explains, "Unlike . . . memorials built by victimized nations and peoples to
themselves . . . those in Germany are necessarily those of the persecutor
remembering its victims" (53).[16] This is clear in the didactic signage citing the convictions, imprisonment, and murder of gay men under the
Nazi regime. The agency of this memorial, as articulated here, is that of
"Germany," which, as a result of this history, "has a special responsibility
to actively oppose the violation of gay men's and lesbians' human rights."
The plaque concludes: "With this memorial, the Federal Republic of Germany intends to honour the victims of persecution and murder, to keep
alive the memory of this injustice, and to create a lasting symbol of opposition to enmity, intolerance and the exclusion of gay men and lesbians."
    There is a striking visual concordance between Dragset and Elm-
green's homage to victims and the proposals Betsky cites of architects'
evocations of "the experience of queer space" by "queer architects try-

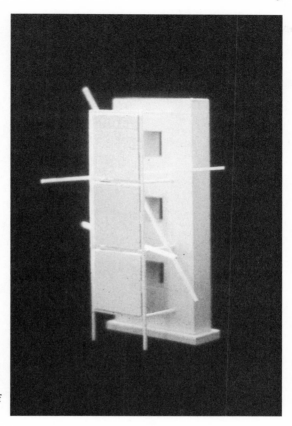

Durham Crout,
model for *Wasting
Architecture,* proposed
AIDS memorial,
prototype realized in
San Francisco, 1993.
Photograph courtesy of
Durham Crout.

ing to make sense out of their world in the age of AIDS" (*Queer Space,*
184–85). The similarity is especially strong between the Berlin monument and Betsky's illustration of part of Durham Crout's 1993 proposal
for a symbolic structure titled *Wasting Architecture* (186).[17] The Berlin
memorial might also be compared to Mark Robbins's *Utopian Prospect,* a
1988 installation on the grounds of the Byrdcliffe Colony in Woodstock,
New York. As staged for Robbins's presentation photographs, the peek-
a-boo windows in this cinderblock wall frame glimpses of actual naked
young men.[18] These proposed and realized monuments share a visual
language that, like many theories of "queer space," pictures gay men (and
all of these monuments are about men) as hidden, isolated, and subject to
a "peeping" gaze.[19] That the same counter-monumental visual language can
seem to speak for the (remorseful) persecutors of gay men or for "queer

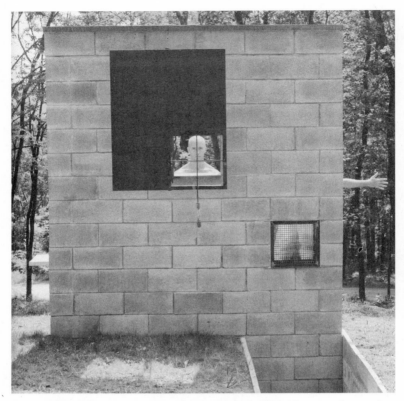

Mark Robbins, *Utopian Prospect,* Woodstock, New York, block, bluestone, glass, steel, 1988. Photograph courtesy of Mark Robbins.

architects" returns us to the critique, articulated in the Introduction, of the way first-wave queer theory valorized the blurring of boundaries between stealth and fear, victim and perpetrator, anger and shame. We return to these issues in chapter 4.

Such conflicted relations to visibility in the era after AIDS stand in striking contrast to the two earlier monuments discussed in this chapter, both commissioned in 1979. For all of their visual differences, these shared an assumption that homosexual identity, as much as any other, deserved its own *lieux de mémoire.* In the crisis of memory that followed the on-slaught of AIDS, however, there was a pulling back from spatial visibility that paralleled calls for the de-generational unremembering of a diseased lifestyle connected to a shameful history. *Lieux de mémoire*, which affirm an identity constructed in the present in relation to the past, become impossible to imagine in the absence of the aspiration to a shared memory that was one of the many casualties of AIDS.

Seeing and Being Seen: Neighborhoods

Like monuments, neighborhoods have gotten short shrift in most queer-theoretical accounts, which set themselves against the idea that sexual identity could find visual expression in the built environment. This blinkered view contrasts with the record of frequent, albeit often condescending, observation by other scholars of the impact of minority sexual culture on the look of neighborhoods. As early as 1976, the influential architectural theorist Charles Jencks cited as a source for "post-modernism" (a term just coming into currency at the time) what he called the "Gay Eclectic" style of extravagantly ornamented exteriors superimposed on run-of-the-mill bungalows "in the lesser side of Beverly Hills." A few years later, Jencks rechristened the style "Boys Town Variegated," but his point remained that the semiotic playfulness of an architectural style associated with gay men played a crucial role in the coup against modernist "puritanical building." Describing the practitioners of Gay Eclectic/Boys Town style as "interior designers who went exterior," Jencks concludes of the results: "Most are cloying; but the language [of architecture] is at least being used (instead of entirely dominating the speaker)."[20] As post-modernism — and Jencks — became more established, references to its gay origins dropped out of later editions of his influential *The Language of Post-Modern Architecture*. Right-wing cultural critics were, of course, happy to condemn all of postmodernism as simply a manifestation of camp, with the reminder that "camp humor derives, in its essence, from the homosexual's recognition that his condition represents a kind of joke on nature, a denial of its imperatives" (Kramer, *The Revenge of the Philistines*, 6). But queer theories of the built environment neither expanded upon Jencks's early citations nor contested the condescending tone of his point that the exaggeration of architectural signifiers he identified as "Gay" was an assertion of control over the dominant visual discourses of suburban domesticity.

Instead of developing the rich possibilities in the idea that sexual identity could find expression in the built environment (and vice versa), when queer theory turned to architecture, it was to continue to insist on invisibility. Betsky asserted, "By its very nature, queer space is something that is not built, only implied, and usually invisible" (*Queer Space*, 18).[21] Sociologists and geographers associated with queer theory reiterated their insistence — even in the face of evidence to the contrary — on the "low visibility" of residential designs for lesbians and gay men.[22] This might have been true at one time and in some instances. In 1973, commentary in an architecture journal bemoaned "the almost total invisibility of gay life in LA" (Usborne, "Gay LA"). Maxine Wolfe's history of lesbian bars and their "people/environment relationships" is titled "Invisible Women in Invisible Places," while another study of gay and lesbian bars in the seventies analyzes their shuttered and camouflaged street façades, mazelike entryways, and intimidating signage as evidence that these spaces "incorporate and reflect certain characteristics of the gay community: secrecy and stigmatization. They do not accommodate the eyes of outsiders, they have low imageability" (Weightman, "Gay Bars as Private Places," 9). But this emphasis ignores the remarkable flowering of queer signs as part of the coming-to-visibility by sexual minorities in the last quarter of the twentieth century. By the 1990s, a souvenir publication from a Lesbian and Gay Pride celebration noted the adaptation of "Queer Street" to "an increasingly confident generation of lesbians and gay men whose sense of Pride means that they want to be visible."[23]

The insistence on the architectural invisibility of queer life runs through analyses of the nature of queer domesticity on the level of both the house and the neighborhood. Of the fourteen projects in the 1994 *Queer Space* exhibition, none proposed a house, and domesticity was framed, in the one project that addressed it, as a site of assimilation so complete as to render queers invisible. For the Family Values project in *Queer Space*, Benjamin Gianni and Mark Robbins asked gays and lesbians in two small cities (Columbus, Ohio, and Ottawa, Ontario) to submit snapshots of their homes in order "to explore (and explode) stereotypes about the gay community, who we are and how we live." The prospectus for the project contrasted images of a house and a gay dance club over a text that extrapolated from the claim that 10 percent of the population is gay to speculate about the whereabouts of the 115,000 "homosexuals" suppos-

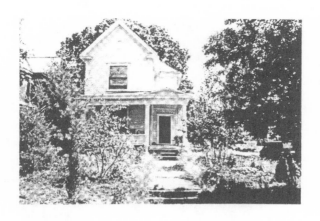

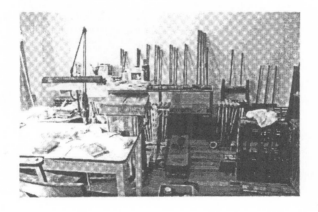

occupancy: two gay men
ages: early forties
dwelling type: house
setting: urban
dependants: two dogs
value of house: $85,000

Benjamin Gianni and Mark Robbins, *Family Values* (detail), photographs and text, 1994.

edly in Columbus but not among the five thousand in the public spaces of "bars, clubs, or cruising areas," and concluded that "the majority of gay people live among their heterosexual neighbors. Some of us react against normative symbols of domesticity, others of us embrace them."[24]

Even a cursory inspection of the photographs submitted for the Family Values project, however, reveals inside the homes depicted characteristics that accord with Jencks's observations concerning Gay Eclectic architecture. Some are extremely high-style. Others recycle unfashionable furnishings in eccentric ways. The snapshot of one gay couple's interior features at least thirty-eight croquet mallets (their profusion makes them hard to count), while the attic bedroom of a lesbian couple is empty but for a bed and a rocking chair holding a large teddy bear.[25] These spaces draw from and extend a history of queer-identified extravagance in domestic design that includes the campy interiors associated with fey interior designers in movies like *Pillow Talk* (1959) and *The Gay Deceivers* (1969), as well as the women's "fantasy drawings" of houses made of domes and swirls, with "retirement and revival circles" and zones for "private strokes and escapes," not to mention subterranean "womb rooms" and air-borne "goddess platforms" where "you can have ice cream or/ and cake and coffee," which were produced in workshops organized in the 1970s by lesbian-feminist activists and architects Leslie Kanes Weisman and Noel Phyllis Birkby.[26] These precedents went unnoted in the presentation of and the critical reaction to the Family Values project, and the installation won favorable reviews for its "de-eroticization of queerness" and concomitant demonstration of the "banality" of gay and lesbian home life (Butler, "Queer Space"). In this view (or failure to view), the invisibility of queerness in the built environment is celebrated as evidence of the triumph of assimilation.

Imperatives to invisibility also structured Gianni's collaborative Queers in (Single-Family) Space house proposal (discussed earlier), which accepted as its premise that "Within the value-laden suburban milieu, difference is accommodated as long as it is kept out of sight." The presentation drawings, done in the campy style of 1950s advertising, introduced the flexible floor plans with headlines like, "That pretty facade hides so much!" and "It may look like a single family house . . . but looks can be deceiving" (Gianni et al., "Queerying (Single-Family) Space" [ellipses in original]). A similar dynamic animates Joel Sanders's 1999 Bachelor House

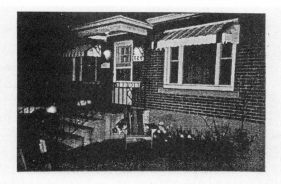

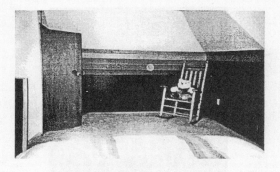

occupants: lesbian with lover	*"My lover is differently abled with vision*
ages: 26 and 33	*and mobility difficulties. Home was*
dwelling type: house	*renovated with her challenges in mind.*
setting: urban	*We are conscious of security, with a*
dependants: a cat and twenty fish	*private fenced yard, deck and security*
household income: $54,000	*system. We love to travel, and would*
value of house: $150,000	*rather spend our money on travel, etc.*
notes: renovated for accessibility	*than a large house."*

project, which, although it was included in the Museum of Modern Art's
The Un-Private House exhibition, was organized around a highly developed sense of privacy. "Built on the foundations of a 1950s Rambler"
ranch, the Bachelor House defers to the established look of its neighborhood while presenting high walls, small windows, and a blank garage

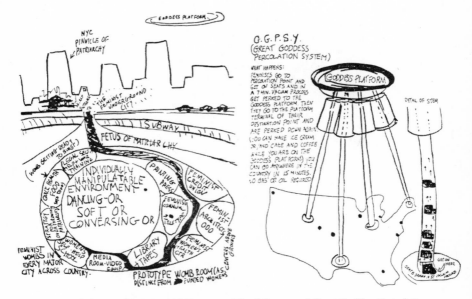

Women's fantasy drawings with Prototype Womb Room and Great Goddess Percolation System, solicited by Phyllis Birkby and Leslie Kanes Weisman, c. 1975. Reproduced from *Quest: A Feminist Quarterly* (Summer 1975).

door to the street in what the architect called "a kind of subterfuge, a kind of camouflage" to protect the "bachelor" within "from the prying eyes of disapproving neighbors."[27]

Our point is not to diminish the creativity of these designs. Much like the extravagant vernacular domestic interiors documented in the Family Values project, the Bachelor House's buttoned-down exterior gives way — rather fabulously through the transparent back wall of the bachelor's garage, where "parking his car...he can see his whole living space through the windshield" — to an interior that plays imaginatively with the erotics of sight.[28] Equally provocative, the covered, sunken Astroturf backyard "out of the neighbors' view" opens into an "underground spa" with a backlit translucent shower, all visible from the master bedroom (Riley 100–101). The problem with the Bachelor House and the Queers in (Single-Family) Space projects — both presented as theoretical paradigms in well-publicized exhibitions at important museums — is not the innovations in their interiors but the uncritical assumption that the look of queerness in the built environment of the neighborhood must be invisibility.

The irony is that this theoretical predilection for queer invisibility emerged in the 1990s at just the time street activists chanting, "We're here! We're queer! Get used to it!" made "visibility" the order of the day. In this regard it is significant that although the presentation of the Bachelor House asserts, "our design responds to our client," when we queried Sanders about this client's ideas about privacy, his first response was to recall that the bachelor was concerned with "concealing unsightly views of neighbors."[29] Like the ACT UP activists who taunted the cops in surgical gloves with "Your hats don't match your shoes!" or the later television series *Queer Eye for the Straight Guy*, this form of queerness was not about hiding or masking but about asserting queerness as a superior form of visual sensitivity. Understood as barriers against looking out, rather than shields against those looking in, the high walls and tiny street-facing windows of the Bachelor House could be read as the architectural expression of the theatrical horror with which *Queer Eye*'s "Fabulous Five" responded to the wardrobes and living rooms of their as-yet unreconstructed straight clients.

The investment of those who theorize the queer-built environment in an ideal of invisibility, however, left the look of queer neighborhoods largely untheorized, although real estate agents and journalists were quick to notice changes to the look of urban neighborhoods when queers moved in, renovations began, "Silence Equals Death" posters popped up in windows, and rainbow flags sprouted on porches and balconies. Nor were theoretical generalizations about the neighbors' hostility always realized in practice (when teenagers stole the rainbow flag from our porch in Portland, Maine, in the mid-1990s, a neighbor we had never met was walking her dog, recognized the flag as it was being borne down the street, took it from the vandals, and returned it to us before we even knew it was missing). In certain neighborhoods in major—and some midsized—cities, the density of pink triangles, equality symbols, and Amazon bumper stickers accumulated to create a collective and vernacular version of the imminence achieved by the *Homomonument*, where an accumulation of individual elements can charge an entire space.

Like Jencks's speculations concerning Gay Eclectic design of individual houses, analyses of the look of gay neighborhoods appeared early on from high-profile scholars, although these were ignored by later theorists. Prominent sociologist Manuel Castells, in his 1983 book *The City and the*

Grassroots, for instance, recognized the distinctive look of the Castro district in San Francisco. Noting that "space is a fundamental dimension of the gay community" (145), Castells described the "careful painting of the original Victorian facades" in the Castro and the "well-designed treatment of semi-public spaces—between the front door and the pavement for example," which stood out to this European viewer as "a very unusual architectural improvement in the highly individualistic world of American cities" (166). Castells analyzed the look of the Castro as an expression of gay sensibility, not in the essentialized way that would become ritualistically denied by queer theorists but as an outcome of social forces. "Gay men," he argued, are the products of

> two processes of socialization. . . . On the one hand, they grow up as men, and therefore are taught to believe in the values of power, conquest, and self-affirmation. . . . At the same time, because of the feelings that many have had to hide for years, and some for their entire life, they develop a special sensitiveness, a desire for communication, a high esteem of solidarity and tenderness that brings them closer to women's culture. This is not, however, because gay men are "feminine," but, like women, their oppression and discrimination create a distance from the values of conquest and domination which they are supposed to share as men. Thus they tend to consider the use value of their personal lives as important, or worth more than the exchange value that could be acquired without ever obtaining the greatest reward of all— to be themselves. And yet power and money still matter for many gay men. The spatial expression of this twofold desire for exchange value and use value is, in our opinion, housing renovation. (166–67)

The conclusion of Castells's analysis is that the dramatically renovated houses of the Castro—and the phenomenon was hardly confined to San Francisco—were, far from being invisible, a way of "saying something to the city while expressing something to its own dwellers. . . . This is perhaps the most important contribution of the gay community to the city: not only housing improvement but urban meaningfulness"(167).[30]

To acknowledge that meaningfulness is there to see is a prerequisite to any analysis of the look of gay neighborhoods. Such meanings are undoubtedly many and various, but we want to emphasize that in the context of the 1970s and early 1980s when "urban renewal" was still overwhelmingly associated with razing and rebuilding, the look of these thriving gay neighborhoods was distinctive for the way it referred to the past. It was not just the "Painted Ladies" of San Francisco, but the art deco low-rises of Miami Beach, the townhouses of Back Bay, the tiny "trinities" around 13th Street in Philadelphia—all of these gay neighborhoods looked treasured not despite their out-of-date aesthetics but because of them.

This renovation aesthetic is not confined to urban areas, although these were where it was initially most visible. Recently, the restoration of distinctive 1950s suburban developments like Atlanta's Northcrest has also been linked to an influx of gay men. Even some quintessentially rural sites—prime among them probably the tiny mining village of Pendarvis, Wisconsin (now a state historic site)—owe their preservation to gay men (Fellows, *A Passion to Preserve*, 191–99). Allan Gurganus's poignantly funny 1994 novella "Preservation News" is cast as an issue of a North Carolina newsletter for historic preservationists, beginning with the last article by its founder, written as he was dying of AIDS, followed by a rambling obituary by one of his devoted dowager volunteers. Of course, rehabilitation also caught on outside gay communities in American cities, but this does not delegitimate the initial widespread observation that it began among gays. Indeed, urban renovation might be counted with disco, earrings on men, and blue jeans as fashion on the list of contributions to the look of contemporary life that originated in the gay community.

It's no great stretch from Castells's analysis to recognize what we might call the pastness of gay neighborhoods as a visual signal of dissent from prevailing social norms. Treasuring aesthetics the dominant culture has rejected as mannered, artificial, corrupted, superfluous has obvious parallels with the determination to embrace a sexual identity dismissed in much the same terms. And the specific ways the past is treasured correlate with aspects of gay culture, in particular "camp," that much-contested but—starting in the 1960s—crucial analytical term, which Esther Newton in 1972 compared to African American "Soul" as a "subcultural ideology" ("Role Models," 46). Susan Sontag's hugely influential "Notes on Camp," first published in 1964, identified "Camp taste" as "a kind of love. . . . It relishes, rather than judges, the little triumphs and awkward intensities of 'character'" (293). Sontag noted camp's attraction to the "old-fashioned, out-of-date, *démodé*" but saw this turn toward the past as incidental: "It's not a love of the old as such. It's simply that the process of aging or deterioration provides the necessary detachment—or arouses the necessary sympathy" (286–87). History is more central to Andrew Ross's important 1989 chapter, "Uses of Camp," which insists that "the camp effect" requires that aspects of "a much earlier mode of production . . . become available, in the present, for redefinition according to contemporary modes of taste" (*No Respect*, 139). Ross and Sontag agree, however, that camp is a generous impulse that counters norms that dismiss or condemn. Quoting Mark Booth's claim that "to be camp is to present oneself as being committed to the marginal with a commitment greater than the marginal merits" (in Ross, 146), Ross notes camp's "pre-Stonewall heyday" as "part of a survivalist culture which found . . . a way of imaginatively communicating its common conquest of everyday oppression" (157). The links between identifications with the past and "survivalist" modes of imaginative invention define the importance of memory to the innovative and renovative continuation of queer culture across—and often despite—time.

The look of camp in the built environment has been—often pejoratively—associated with the postmodern turn toward anachronistic, overscale ornamentation that Jencks first identified on the "Gay Eclectic" houses of West Hollywood in the 1970s and that Philip Johnson made famous with the Chippendale-topped AT&T building in Manhattan completed in 1984 (known officially since 1992 as the Sony Tower). Certainly analyzable in Sontag's terms as an awkwardly intense invocation of the old-fashioned, the AT&T building made unmissable camp tendencies long present in Johnson's architecture. Referring to some of Johnson's 1960s designs, the architectural historian Andrew Saint wrote a bitterly homophobic obituary that derided "the camp arches of his so-called ballet-school style" ("Philip Johnson"). Looking back further, and more admiringly, another historian, Alice Friedman, takes seriously the camp effects of the Glass House, which Johnson built on his Connecticut estate in 1949. Noting that "gay men and lesbians" at midcentury "developed a rich 'underground' culture of their own," Friedman values camp, with its "heavy emphasis on irony, exaggeration, artifice, and of course humor," as both a protective buffer against "heterosexual culture" and a way to "cast doubt on the whole weighty, self-sustaining system of gender roles, social norms, and conventional appearances." She reads the Glass House—an open living space around a brick column that contains a fireplace (and conceals a tiny bathroom) — as "an obvious and clearly ironic reference to the architecture of the traditional American family home and to the sentimentalized view of domesticity that had gained widespread currency since the late nineteenth century." The openness of this gay man's weekend retreat where Johnson "entertained gay friends from New York at elegant cocktail parties and dinners" stands in marked contrast to the nearby Guest House, which "appears to be a windowless bunker, a defensible place of intimacy as well as a 'closet'. . . . Like the nondescript gay bars of the period, it turns its back on its surroundings" (*Women and the Making,* 152–53).

Friedman's subtle reading invokes both history (the implied contrast with nineteenth-century domestic paradigms) and visibility (the openness of the Glass House in comparison with the Guest House) to analyze the subversive power of Johnson's architectural rhetoric. More typically, the Glass House is classified as deferential (to Mies van der Rohe's glass architecture) and impotent: a unique tour-de-force (or self-indulgence) with little relevance to the development of American domestic architecture. This last claim overlooks the fact that, since the popularization of loft architecture during the 1980s, millions of Americans live in spaces that echo the architectural language of the Glass House: expansive wall-less, doorless spaces defined by exposed girders and plate glass windows. From the beginning, the loft aesthetic explicitly invoked the past, as designers left exposed brick walls and built-in industrial components to speak not only to the anticonventionality of these domestic spaces but to the taste for the outmoded associated with camp.

Unsurprisingly, loft living was also associated with gay neighborhoods — the kinds of spaces "artists" moved into — and with specific gay architects, most notably Alan Buchsbaum, whose own influential 1976 loft (which appeared in the *New York Times* in 1977) featured a bedroom separated from the living space by an undulating barrier of glass brick and a doorless bathroom with an open shower. "The pre-AIDS seventies — free love, open sex, gay discos, the New York baths scene — was the context for Buchsbaum's own laboratory-for-design lofts and their programs for almost-public baths in private spaces," explains his colleague, Frederick Schwartz, who notes, "What looks common in Buchsbaum's work today was then daring and unorthodox" (*Alan Buchsbaum, Architect and Designer,* 14, 11). Like the restoration aesthetic, the renovation aesthetic manifest in the domestic lofts ubiquitous today may make it difficult to recognize the subcultural origins of their characteristic elements, but these are crucially related to the visual emphasis on the past in the juxtaposition of new—glass brick, high-tech lighting and kitchen appliances—and old that is a signature of loft design. Pioneering the look that came to define urban lofts, Buchsbaum retained the original tin ceilings, hardwood floors, exposed joists, and patches of brick in the nineteenth-century light-industrial spaces he rehabbed, explaining, "I find pleasure in seeing the rough quality of existing construction contrasted with shiny new materials" (71). Like beard stubble poking through the pancake makeup of a drag queen, the juxtapositions in Buchsbaum's collage aesthetic "play with and question . . . the notion of the real," as he put it (10).

Gay neighborhoods, then, beginning at least from the 1970s, manifested specific forms of visibility through a combination of overt symbols (pink triangles and later rainbow flags, political posters, bumper stickers, graffiti) and a campy architectural style centered on the past (rehabbed lofts, renovated houses in styles gone by, or, often, some combination). We argue further that the pastness of these neighborhoods extended beyond the look of buildings, creating—or reflecting—forms of social life that were considered "old-fashioned, out-of-date, *démodé*" once planners started organizing urban spaces around automobiles. The high density of storefront and housefront display in gay neighborhoods, however, corresponded with unusually dense pedestrian traffic even in cities that were otherwise automobile-based and at times when other areas were deserted. This passage could describe queer districts in any number of American or European cities in the 1990s, though its referent is farther afield:

> While most of downtown Johannesburg is deserted by six or seven in the evening, Hillbrow stays open all night. There are sidewalk cafés, book and record shops, movie theatres, and Indian and Near Eastern restaurants. Vendors hawking sandstone hippos and wooden sculpture set up shop on sidewalks" (Miller, *Out in the World*, 13).

On a more somber note, Simon Watney has described how, in London and New York, spontaneous memorials to individuals lost to AIDS turned up along the sidewalks and in the shop windows and cafés of gay neighborhoods: "This is how communities communicate, how the streets talk eloquently about those who passed along them," he concludes (*Imagine Hope*, 167).

The pedestrian attraction (dare we say *pedephilia?*) of gay neighborhoods extends another historical legacy, that of the flâneur, the late-nineteenth-century urban wanderer closely allied with the "dandy" and with promiscuous male sexuality, although Sally Munt traces a corollary heritage of the "lesbian flâneur" from the transvestite George Sand, through Djuna Barnes and Renée Vivien, to Joan Nestle and Sarah Schulman ("The Lesbian Flâneur," 117–21). Although the figure of the flâneur was invoked by Jean-Ulrick Désert (quoted in the introduction to this chapter) as the exemplary queer actor who temporarily queers the space she or he occupies, his emphasis on performance overlooks what made the flâneur, in the era of Impressionism, the paradigm for the modern painter: the flâneur is, above all, a good looker, someone who strolls the sidewalks attentive to what the visual aspect of people and places reveals about the city and its inhabitants, and who records those sights in painting or in prose. In contrast, the exhortations to invisibility embedded in much queer theorizing of the urban (and suburban) environment bespeak not simply an empirical failure to see but a campaign of unremembering waged against acknowledging the fanciful, emotionally invested, sentimental engagement with the past that is characterized by the term camp and visually characteristic of queer neighborhoods.

Neighborhoods as Monuments/Monuments for Neighborhoods

Tensions between imperatives to forget and to remember, between desires for invisibility and the urge to demarcate queer space, played out dramatically in a controversy that roiled Chicago in the late 1990s when the city proposed a project that constituted at least two firsts: the first government-funded marker of minority sexual identity (both the *Homomonument* and *Gay Liberation* were privately funded, although some governments gave some money to the *Homomonument* fund drive) and the first attempt to deploy the visual vocabulary of monuments to signify a queer space larger than the scale of an urban square, that is, to designate an entire neighborhood.

This still-surprising initiative shocked the local merchants' association when emissaries from Mayor Richard M. Daley's office first proposed the project in the summer of 1997 (one informant reported assuming they had been called together to be berated — again — about noise and mess on the sidewalks outside the bars). It provoked news coverage as far away as New York, Washington, San Diego, and London. And it certainly aroused the public, which—encouraged by right-wing, evangelical churches nationwide—sent over seven thousand pieces of mail to the city, more than had ever been generated about any other proposed project, most of it vehemently hostile to the project (this was the era when Pat Robertson, on the Christian Broadcasting Network's *700 Club,* warned that Orlando, Florida, risked hurricanes and the rest of the nation risked terrorist bombing, earthquakes, and/or a meteor for flying Gay Pride flags).[31]

All politics is local, as Tip O'Neill famously remarked, and there was a local backstory for this project: Chicago had recently installed distinctive, custom-designed street markers in its "Chinatown" and "Greektown," as well as in a Puerto Rican neighborhood, all as part of an effort to recast—in the eyes of its own residents, those who had fled to the suburbs, and tourists—the "problem" of the city's racial and ethnic diversity as a source of pride and a magnet for visitors.[32] For the Greektown and Chinatown projects, city designers created pavilions and patterned sidewalks that marked the urban fabric with allusions to ethnically specific architecture (temples and spires for Greektown, pagodas for Chinatown) and symbolic motifs (Greek keys and Chinese dragons). More ambitiously, the mayor hired the prominent architect Edward Windhorst to design two monumental gateway structures for the Puerto Rican neighborhood around Humboldt Park. The Puerto Rican Gates, as they came to be known, drew on motifs from the Puerto Rican flags that struck Windhorst as ubiquitous in the neighborhood.[33] Once installed in 1995, his design was enthusiastically received by the local community, commended by the architectural establishment, and published in the national art press.[34] Following this success, the mayor, in the summer of 1997, commissioned Windhorst to design markers for North Halsted Street in another distinctive Chicago neighborhood, one that real estate agents called Lakeview but everyone else knew as Boys Town.

Following the paradigm that had worked for the Puerto Rican Gates, Windhorst began by visiting the neighborhood. "I walked through the North Halsted area to find out how gays represent themselves. And overwhelmingly what I saw in shop windows, on car bumpers, and in the air were rainbow flags, so rainbow stripes became my theme for the project," he said, explaining the rings of colored LED lights featured in his original design (in Mohr, "Architects of Identity"). Windhorst, who is not gay (or Puerto Rican), was also struck by other distinctive visual characteristics of gay neighborhoods. His original design featured, along the street between two abstract gateway structures, a parade of nearly two hundred large, rainbow-ringed, illuminated pylons that clearly responded to the pedestrian-centered nighttime culture of the neighborhood.

In the ensuing controversy, these elements were critiqued in rhetorics where homophobia lurked either on or close to the surface. A columnist in the *Chicago Sun-Times,* mocking the reification of gay identity in urban design, sarcastically imagined its complement:

> [The city] also needs to celebrate a neighborhood for its heterosexuality.... To avoid confusion, though, the kind of twinkling "rainbow rings of lights" that will adorn the tops of the Boys Town pylons will have to go. Replaced I suppose with likenesses of Ozzie and Harriet. Only straight sidewalks would be permitted. (Byrne, "Everybody on Board")

As is often the case when members of a dominant class imagine they are satirizing demands for "special" recognition from minorities, this purported fantasy of straight-identified space is not far from reality. In addition to the ubiquitous presence of "Ozzie and Harriet"–type images across public spaces throughout Chicago (and beyond), this attempt at parody is close to a paraphrase of an 1869 guide to the Chicago area that described suburban Evanston, known for its religiosity and strict temperance laws, as "laid out at right angles, as rigidly as Methodism itself could demand."[35] Quotations in the gay press from self-identified gay people reflected an internalized homophobia framed as an aversion to display: "I just think those lights and stuff are gaudy. I mean, if I were them *[sic],* the city or the merchant's association or whomever *[sic]* decided to do this, I would at least consider the possibility that people would be scared away from the neighborhood.... the less ostentatious queers, as well as the straights."[36] Pejorative associations with the most overt visual manifestations of gay culture — camp and drag — permeated critiques of the design. The *Chicago Tribune* quoted neighborhood residents at a community meeting complaining that the design was "taking Halsted and putting it in drag" and "over the top" (in Frisch, "Gay-Pride Theme"). By the same token, articles with headlines like "'Gay Pride' Street Markers Get a Toning Down" (Tucker) and "Gay Theme Toned Down in Halsted St. Plan" (Banchero) used terms like "more subtle," "less gaudy," and "more refined" to describe changes in the plan following the period of public debate.

The project as built is a diminished version of the exuberant original proposal. The gateway structures were eliminated, and the number of pylons shrank to twenty-two, now positioned in the middle of each block so as not to be visible from the residential side streets from which the most vociferous local objections emerged. The rainbows of colored lights were replaced by painted bands, "dramatically uplit from the bottom for nighttime effect, but . . . largely neutral in the daylight," as the Department of Transportation's (DOT) prospectus put it, although even this is an exaggeration, as the light from the small white floodlights in each pylon is engulfed by the glow from the taller and much brighter streetlights. What remains as a signifier, in addition to the fact of the rainbow bands, is an architecture that strikes viewers as strangely out of time, at once futuristic and nostalgic. The pylons have been compared, with justice, to both "rocket ships" and to the art deco Chrysler Building in New York (Engelbrecht, "North Halsted Streetscape Plans 'Set'"). "Futuristic metal shafts," "Buck Rogers–style rainbow shafts" (Mohr, "Architects of Identity"), "space-age steel pylons" (Savage, "The Metropolis Observed"), and "Art Deco pylons" (Smallwood, "Gay-Pride Halsted Street Project") were some of the terms journalists used to characterize the elements that the DOT prospectus called "identity columns." These evocations of the high-style futuristic fantasies of the past seem an appropriate marker of a gay neighborhood in the context of the other projects that combine flag imagery with architecture evocative of the past (temples and pagodas) to cast ethnic identity in the streetscape of contemporary Chicago.

The idea of a homeland elsewhere is, of course, central to diasporic ethnic identity, an association the classicist Daniel Mendelsohn appropriates for "queer space" when he suggests that gay neighborhoods, misnamed "ghettos," might more accurately be called *apoikiai*, the Greek word for "colonies" that means "away-from-homes" (*The Elusive Embrace*, 29). But geographical distance merges with — and is ultimately subsumed in — temporal distance as ethnically identified populations establish themselves in an adopted land. In nostalgia for the "old country," the emphasis is on the "old" in the memory of the migrant who recalls a place in

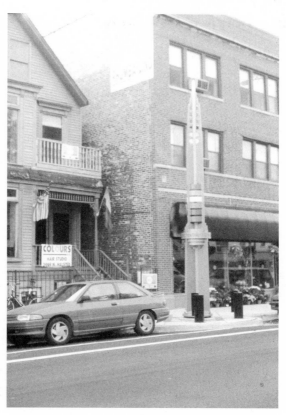

Element of North
Halsted Streetscape
project, Edward
Windhorst, designer;
dedicated 1998. Photo-
graph by Christopher
Reed, 1999.

the past, a place that may no longer exist, and certainly no longer exists
as she or he remembers it. This emphasis on the past is even stronger
among second- or third- (or more) generation ethnics, whose identification rests on imaginative associations with the places their parents or
grandparents came from and often extends to the "old neighborhood"
in a new-world inner city. Fantasies of the past also animate the "new
ethnicity," identified by sociologists as an increasingly important aspect
of global culture in which people, for reasons ranging from marriage
into an ethnic group to a desire to "disaggregate" or "deassimilate" from
dominant social and commercial norms, self-consciously adopt ethnic
identities in midlife (Epstein, "Gay Politics, Ethnic Identity," 84). Steven
Epstein's influential 1987 essay, "Gay Politics, Ethnic Identity: The Limits
of Social Constructionism," highlights the importance of will and fantasy

in constructions of ethnic identity as part of his strategy to transcend paralyzing debates between essentialist and social-construction models of sexual identity by showing that accepted notions of ethnicity managed to include *both* biology and culture (the divisiveness of these debates in relation to sexual identity exemplifies the inequitable scrutiny, alluded to in the introduction to this section, that is focused on claims concerning sexual—as opposed to ethnic, regional, or national—forms of identity). One implication of Epstein's powerful argument is that viable notions of sexual identity require the sense of pastness that ethnic identities assume as their basis.

To return to the ideas proposed in the opening of this chapter, *lieux de mémoire*—places of memory—play an important role in creating and sustaining the invested sense of history that is memory. As long as there has been homosexual identity, this desire for history has been expressed as a yearning for a lost sense of place. Victorians often cast the long-lost queer homeland as ancient Greece. The first edition of John Addington Symonds's 1873 *Studies of the Greek Poets,* a foundational text of homosexual identity, offered the assertion (so provocative that it was omitted from later editions): "Some will always be found . . . to whom Greece is a lost fatherland, and who, passing through youth with the *mal du pays* of that irrecoverable land upon them, may be compared to visionaries" (2:422). This sense of queerness as Greekness found occasional architectural expression in neoclassical "temples of friendship," inspired by Voltaire's poem of that name, which describes a structure dedicated to the same-sex couples of antiquity whose ideal of pure love is contrasted to baser modern desires associated with worldly ambition and heterosexual passion. As early as 1768, Frederic II of Prussia erected on the grounds of his palace near Potsdam one such temple, its columns ornamented with carved medallions depicting male couples (Vogtherr, "Absent Love," 81–82). A similar temple, its pediment inscribed with "A L'AMITIE" ("to friendship"), graced Natalie Barney's garden in Paris, where it became the center of Sapphic celebration during the early twentieth century (Rodriguez, *Wild Heart, A Life,* 175).

In the context of contemporary cities, however, it may be best to leave Greektown to the Greeks. For those trying to visualize the place of queer identity in an urban context where ethnicity is marked by the flags and architectural styles of a homeland, the challenge presents itself in the form of a question about the past: Where did queers come from? Though the Chrysler Building profile of the Boys Town pylons might hint that our homeland is Manhattan, the multicolored rings and over-the-top fantasy of this procession of elements suggest another city, one somewhere over the rainbow, in a land that we've heard of . . . where art deco is the indigenous architectural idiom. And that may not be a bad guess, at least not in a symbolic economy where Chinese Americans come from pagodas and Greek Americans from Corinthian temples. If, as Chicago's other urban markers assert, ethnic identity is constituted in relation to a fantasy/memory of a realm elsewhere, why not choose Oz—and, by inference, the whole glamorous bygone world of midcentury Hollywood—as the gay homeland? Indeed, if Arjun Appadurai is right to argue that traditional forms of ethnic identity have been replaced by "diasporic public spheres" created through electronic media, the location of an originary gay homeland in film confirms Epstein's arguments about the convergence of sexuality and ethnicity as social formations.

Imagining a gay origin-place in Oz may be particularly appropriate to Chicago, where the White City of the 1893 Columbian Exposition inspired L. Frank Baum to imagine the Emerald City. Baum's Chicago roots are commemorated at Oz Park, not far from Boys Town, where, since 1995, sculptor John Kearney's monumental Tin Man has stood on a piazza of yellow bricks inscribed with the names of donors, among whom—in another visual marker of the neighborhood's demographics—are some same-sex couples. Links between gay identity and *The Wizard of Oz* extend beyond the history of Chicago, however. To be a "friend of Dorothy's" is a long-standing euphemism for male homosexuality, and we are hardly the first to note contemporary gay culture's connection to the 1939 camp movie classic starring Judy Garland. This chapter concludes, therefore, by exploring the appeal of this film in relation to our ideas about the importance of place in constructing memory as a mode of collective and revisionary invention in the present, rather than a transparent recuperation of the past.

"There's no place like home!" Dorothy's ambivalent mantra simultaneously asserts and denies the power of nostalgic memory in a pithy encapsulation of the plot of this famous film, in which the heroine's misery in emotionally parched rural America (a paradigmatic trope of many "coming out" stories) is transformed by her fantastical migration to Oz.[37]

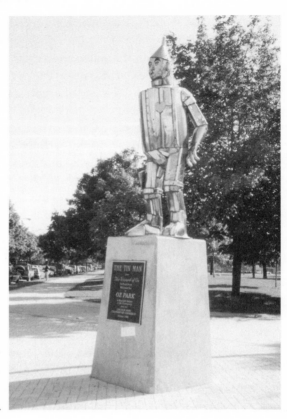

John Kearney, *Tin Man,*
Oz Park, Chicago,
1995. Photograph by
Christopher Reed, 1998.

As she first encounters it, Oz is overtly—if confusingly—ethnicized as
the half-African, half-Bavarian Munchkinland, where beehive-shaped,
wattle-roofed huts, neatly whitewashed and decorated with gingerbread
trim, disgorge miniature inhabitants dressed for an Oktoberfest in what
seems an unwitting parody of the parade of ethnic villages along the
Midway leading to the White City. For Dorothy, Munchkinland's spectacle of ethnicity originates a quest for the gleaming art deco towers of
the Emerald City, where even the horses are rainbow-hued. Dorothy's
successful negotiation of Oz's multiculturalism is grounded in her own
diasporic nostalgia ("I'm Dorothy Gale from Kansas!" she tells everyone
she meets). Back in Kansas, however, her equally powerful memories of
Oz redeem her drab home with roseate—along with all the other hues in
the Technicolor spectrum—memories of Oz. "It was a place!" Dorothy

exclaims when she wakes up on the farm and looks around her assembled community, "And you, and you, and you, and you were there!" As Salman Rushdie, a critic highly attuned to issues of migration and identity, concluded in his analysis of the film, it is about the "dream of *leaving*.... the real secret of the ruby slippers is not that 'there's no place like home,' but rather that there is no longer any such place *as* home: except, of course, for the home we make, or the homes that are made for us, in Oz: which is anywhere, and everywhere, except the place from which we began" (*The Wizard of Oz*, 23, 57).

The Wizard of Oz represents the formation of what recent scholarship on ethnicity calls the "third cultures" that expatriates create by synthesizing the ideals and images of a homeland into the culture of their host countries (Featherstone). Dorothy Gale, mediating between the urban ethnic hodgepodge of Oz and the monoculture of the homeland, personifies the status of "new ethnicities" in America's modernizing cities. Rarely recognized in such accounts of third cultures, however, are the neighborhoods created and marked by sexual minorities, although one of the most remarkable accomplishments of late-twentieth-century gay culture has been the purposeful reanimation of the spaces and institutions of diasporic urban culture that sociologists and urban planners at midcentury confidently dismissed as doomed to extinction. Moving like Dorothy from rural America to urban centers (and sometimes, also like her, back again), gays and lesbians, following ways of life associated with the liminality of immigration, enacted dissent from the homogenizing effects of the heteronormative melting pot, a dissent that found visual expression in the overtly anachronistic. Part "new ethnicity," part camp, these reparative efforts created spaces of protection and expression, at once old and avant-garde, bounded but permeable, distinguished from mainstream culture by both temporal and spatial displacements.

In her use of memory to supplement and revise the shortcomings of whatever location she finds herself in, Dorothy Gale personifies a subtle addendum to Pierre Nora's theories of *lieux de mémoire*. It is not simply that place is central to the recollections of memory; memory is also central to our capacity to adapt to, reimagine, and revise our places. If memory were simply transparent recollection, Dorothy need never have left Oz; she could have simply "remembered" Kansas into her new home. But memory was not, for her, a mode of recuperation—how could it be, when the "home" she remembers is "no place" (there's no place like home)? Memory, for Dorothy, is, rather, a psychic buffer-zone, a space of distance from the present that allows her to interpret and re-imagine her way to greater satisfaction. That satisfaction arises in part from an awareness that memories are contagious: Dorothy's nostalgic longing for Kansas awakens in her companions in Oz similar longings (for brains, courage, etc.). Memory and desire, collapsing time and hybridizing space, alienating homelands but creating new forms of belonging, become, for Dorothy, both collectivizing and transformative. It is fitting, then, that Dorothy became an icon for gay culture, similarly located in the spatial and temporal interstices of memory and invention.

"*Lieux de mémoire* originate," Nora wrote, "with the sense that there is no spontaneous memory, that we must deliberately create archives, maintain anniversaries, organize celebrations, pronounce eulogies, and notarize bills because such activities no longer occur naturally" ("Between Memory and History," 12). Perhaps they never did. "Natural" memory might be as flat and featureless as Dorothy's black-and-white home on the plains. Memory, as Nora suggests, takes work, and that is the work undertaken by queers who design monuments, spray-paint rocks, restore houses, create and circulate memory narratives. All are forms of making places for and of memory, especially important at a time when intellectual suspicions — of identity, of collectivity, of marked environments — make the collectivizing work of culture harder to recognize, much less appreciate. We can never live without memory as individuals, or we would cease to have consciousness. We might just as easily cease to have social consciousness without the forms of vernacular memory associated with neighborhoods, monuments, and other markers of collective memory. If we understand the incompleteness or fabrication of those memories as invitations to collective invention in the present rather than as proof of their inadequacy, we might begin to recognize the need for the collectivities organized by memory to have places to meet, create, and encode not only their experiences in the past but their aspirations for the present and future.

3. THE REVOLUTION MIGHT BE TELEVISED

The Mass Mediation of Gay Memories

"In the Real World": Popular Culture and Its Discontents

The preceding chapters explored manifestations of gay memory in independent film and video, in novels, and in the architectural fabric of urban monuments and neighborhoods. Although, as we argue, these manifestations of memory have gone largely overlooked critically, they are nevertheless clearly imbricated within broader dynamics of gay and queer cultures. To turn now to network television is to plunge into more hostile territory. Television has been theorized as among the "apparatuses" that have been "set up . . . to obstruct the flow of . . . popular memory," with reference to the history of "popular struggle" against nationalism, war, and economic exploitation (Foucault, "Film and Popular Memory," 91, 102). Foucault's words are from a 1974 interview in which he contrasted the regime of forgetting enforced by movies, television, and academic curricula with "working class" memories that were "more clearly formulated in the 19th century, where, for instance, there was a tradition of struggles which were transmitted orally, or in writings or songs, etc." (91). George Lipsitz has similarly argued that "the power apparatuses of contemporary commercial electronic mass communications" play an especially invidious role in undermining "the elements of historical inquiry and explanation" embodied in, for example, performances of "spirituals, blues, and jazz" passed down to contemporary African Americans by their "ancestors" (*Time Passages,* 4).

We see television, however, as extending exactly the gender-bending dynamics Lipsitz analyzes in nineteenth-century commercial theater, which, in his words, "emerged in part as a rebellion against sexual repression," creating "a kind of free space for the imagination — an arena liberated from old restraints and repressions, a place where desire did not have to be justified or explained" (9) in conventional gendered terms, so that "women especially utilized the new popular culture as a way of escaping parental surveillance and patriarchal domination" (8). Lipsitz's analysis usefully corrects romantic images of historical continuity passed down in some unproblematically authentic way through folk songs and festivals, weddings and funerals. What shimmers from one perspective as a roseate image of class solidarity looks from another vantage point like patriarchal coercion. Theorists applying queer and feminist perspectives to thinking about the historical development of identities that contest patriarchal norms have cautioned against familial metaphors, especially the idea of "generations," for the way they import assumptions about dynamics of begetting and — in the Freudian model — rebelling (Roof, "Generational Difficulties"). As an alternative to familial paradigms for the perpetuation of memory, we might look to Lipsitz's descriptions of how television — "a 'close-up' medium whose dramatic and social locus is the home" — "intervenes in family relations" with an "illusion of intimacy" that powerfully "addresses the inner life" (*Time Passages,* 18–19) in order to understand how television might be particularly effective in shaping subjectivities associated with minority sexuality and gender rather than with the normative family.

The roots of televised dramas and comedies lie in nineteenth-century forms of "commercialized leisure" that, Lipsitz says, "helped reshape cultural memory and consciousness" (8). Traditional rituals of communal memory were supplanted by "theater attendance," which "enabled individuals to play out fictive scenarios of changed identities, to escape from the surveillance and supervision of moral authorities and institutions" (8). Lipsitz asserts that theatrical role-playing "suggested identities could be changed" and that "theatrical 'time' presented an alternative to work time," encouraging "audiences to pursue personal desires and passions" in a forum where "theatergoers . . . shared intimate and personal cultural moments with strangers" (7–8).

The same historical forces that replaced "the wedding celebration or the community festival" with commercial theater — increasing social and geographic mobility, rapid urbanization, and higher levels of disposable incomes — helped generate modern gay culture (D'Emilio, "Capitalism and Gay Identity"). Sexual identity is not Lipsitz's interest.[1] But his analysis of the dynamics of theater and television suggests close ties with emergent gay culture, which often took shape in the commercial spaces of popular entertainment and shared its constitutive features, so much so that the playwright Neil Bartlett claims, "The history of mainstream entertainment is the history of gay culture" (in Burston, "Just a Gigolo?" 120). Particularly relevant is commercial entertainment's yoking of collective memory and anonymity, in contrast to older forms of remembering that assume unmediated and intimate memory (of family, of village) as the basis of identity. The mass media allow large audiences to share intimacy without familiarity and to create new memories — and hence identities — from seemingly impersonal and specularized encounters (in this regard, earlier mass media prefigured the current Internet sexual culture). As Elizabeth Freeman observes, the capacity of "various culture industries to produce shared subjectivities that go beyond the family" has just begun to be explored ("Packing History, Count(er)ing Generations," 729). Lipsitz's description of the dynamics of popular theater — "The unfamiliarity of the crowd with each other provided a kind of protective cover — a 'privacy in public' whereby personal feelings and emotions could be aired without explanation or apology" (*Time Passages*, 8) — echoes recent historical analysis of sexual subcultures, which has challenged stereotypes of both an exclusively heterosexual "public" and the isolated gloom of the "closet" by showing how queer counterpublics manifested both anonymity and community, secrecy and collective code-making.[2]

Of course, twenty-first-century television is not nineteenth-century popular theater. Many critics of television argue that its potential to subvert dominant social formations or to propose powerful alternatives is severely limited — if not entirely foreclosed — by the advertizing that makes networks answerable to their corporate sponsors. This point is well worth heeding. In the following discussion of *Will and Grace*, we do not deny the limitations imposed by sponsorship on what the show could or could not depict (there are no sex scenes, for instance), nor would we contest that the depiction of gay life in the sitcom privileges white, upper-middle-class urbanites with large disposable incomes. It would be naïve to claim that sitcoms like *Will and Grace,* whatever other subjectivities they may endorse, do not also seek to interpellate viewers into the pleasures of commodity consumption and upward mobility, especially when those economic systems are represented as intrinsically related to sexual pleasure.

At the same time, we also want to resist assuming, as many scholars seem to, that television's investment in capitalism precludes any other cultural work. It is wrong to assume that narratives interpellate in only one ideological register or that viewers will respond to the hail of capital in predictable or compliant ways. Nor should we assume that alternative forms of culture (including avant-garde art and academic criticism) are *not* sponsored by capital. As we note in our discussion of E. P. Thompson in the introduction, we'd be hard-pressed to name a current form of what he called "human occasion" that is not invested in capital. The possibilities of such occasions arise, as Thompson knew, from *within* the commodity, not outside it. For these reasons, we believe that today's mass entertainment, including television, is worth exploring for forms of sexual world-making that would include those people on whose behalf critics fret and whose pleasures they dismiss.

Perhaps the easiest television format to dismiss is the situation comedy, but it is that genre that has had the closest links to nonnormative intimacy and identity. Humor offers an alibi for the depiction of all manner of nonnormative affiliations and ideologies. In the 1970s, Norman Lear's hit series, including *All in the Family, Maude,* and *The Jeffersons,* famously troubled dominant attitudes toward race, gender, class, and war.[3] Even before these overtly political sitcoms, shows like *My Three Sons* and *Green Acres* visualized certain queer possibilities. The three sons of Fred MacMurray demonstrated more about male intimacy, with the help of gruff Uncle Charlie, than almost any show on television, while Hooterville was inhabited by a fashion-crazy drag-wannabe, a female carpenter who always wore her tool belt loaded, several elderly gentlemen who lived alone, and a man in love with a pig. Sitcoms' fascination with nonnormative or chosen families from *I Dream of Jeannie* and *The Courtship of Eddie's Father* through *The Brady Bunch* to *Cheers* and *Friends* suggests a generic linkage between these comedies typically set — and viewed — in the home and fascination with self-motivated, collectively maintained forms of alternative domestic affiliation. More broadly, the seriality of the sitcom format, flexible and prone to revision, subordinates presumptions of identity as unchanging historical fact to more playfully malleable and self-willed paradigms. Sitcoms, by presenting sympathetic, recurring characters whose eccentric misreadings of their environments constitute the primary pleasure of the genre (Eva Gabor's Lisa Douglas in *Green Acres*, Uncle Martin on *My Favorite Martian*, and all the characters except — tellingly — the Professor on *Gilligan's Island*), validated strategies of nonnormative interpretation that are a hallmark of subculture.

Twentieth-century American comedy, as even the most mainstream journalism now acknowledges, has been profoundly shaped by Jewish and gay sensibility (Kirby, "The Boys," 23, 33). It took a long time, however, before these identities could be acknowledged and even longer before television comedies could be frankly situated in these minority communities. *Rhoda* in the mid-1970s offered a pioneering depiction of Jewish community in many ways comparable to the effect, for sexual minorities, of *Will and Grace*, the first television show to invoke gay community by featuring in central roles recurring gay characters (not simply one homosexual stranded in a sea of straightness). The links between *Rhoda* and *Will and Grace* are hinted at in an episode in Season 4, when Grace balks at asking her boyfriend to marry her, and Will, to encourage her, says, "Grace, in the real world, women ask men all the time. Rhoda asked Joe."[4] Like so many lines in *Will and Grace* — like camp in general — this remark is wiser than it first seems. The alibi of comedy has allowed sitcoms sometimes to reflect and revise "the real world" in ways that other television formats have not.[5]

This is not to claim that the treatment of sexual minorities on sitcoms — or on television in general — has been uniformly, or even usually, admirable. On the contrary, a large body of criticism documents the suppression and denigration of homosexuality on television right up to the present. For the 2009–10 season, the Gay & Lesbian Alliance Against Defamation (GLAAD) concluded that just 3 percent of scripted characters in primetime television series could be categorized as LGBT, a figure that, small as it is, doubles the number from 2006 ("GLAAD Study"). But criticism focused on counting characters or on scrutinizing sitcom plotlines and character development for stereotypes misses some fundamental points about the ways comedy works to, among other things, convey memory and, through it, to enable strong identifications with minority sexualities. Such critical methods seem likely to be counterproductive in the face of the particular sensibility known as camp, which is defined by, to quote Susan Sontag, "the love of the exaggerated . . . of things-being-what-they-are-not" ("Notes on Camp," 280). A few years out from 2006, there may be twice the number of queer characters on television, but it's hard to feel they have twice the impact of the final season, in that year, of *Will and Grace*. Making explicit the links between camp and comedy at the same time that it exploited the parallels between gay identity and the viewing logic of popular entertainment, *Will and Grace* realized the sitcom's potential to both reflect and create a "real world" of sexual subculture deeply rooted in the dynamics of gay memory.

Popularity makes a sitcom especially suspicious critically, and few shows in recent memory have been as suspect as *Will and Grace*, which was the surprise hit of 1998, first among gay audiences and then among audiences as a whole.[6] Between 2001 and 2005, it became the highest rated sitcom for adults ages 18 to 49, and during its eight-year history, *Will and Grace* and its actors won several awards sponsored by GLAAD (this in addition to sixteen Emmys).[7] Even a hasty review of the show's episodes, its chatrooms, and existing criticism reveals a dynamic Lipsitz notes as a problem for the study of television in general: that its many detractors, eager to register their perceptions of aesthetic or ideological shortcomings, fail to account for the fact that a significant number of viewers voluntarily watch the show again and again. When these viewers — and their pleasures — are not simply ignored, they tend to be pathologized as manifestations of brainwashing, whether by "the gay agenda" (for the Christian right)[8] or capitalism (for the Marxist left) or (among film theorists) some form of false consciousness following the paradigm of Laura Mulvey's influential characterization of the sadomasochistic pleasures of women socialized to enjoy the spectacle of their own humiliation.[9]

In a dynamic that has been criticized by Edward Schiappa, professional critics, mainly academics, condemned *Will and Grace* for (in the words of one critical article) "reinforcing heterosexism" by "feminizing" its gay characters and failing to "represent a challenge to the dominant norms of U.S. culture"[10] and (in the words of another article) making "the comedic structure of gay bashing . . . central to its rhetorical appeals."[11] As Schiappa notes, these analyses enact a rhetoric of professionalism that allows credentialed critics to distinguish themselves by providing readings "*different* from the sort of descriptions that might be produced by the 'typical' or 'average' viewer." Schiappa continues: "The more radically different a critic's description of a text is from the dominant reading from mainstream culture the better, because the more unusual and distinctive the description, the more clear it is what the 'added value' [of] a particular critic's contribution is. The problem is that the need to produce unusual and distinctive descriptions can encourage a 'trained incapacity' that leads the critic to miss the cultural and political work a text may perform among the general population" (*Beyond Representational Correctness*, 64–65).[12] Schiappa uses *Will and Grace* to frame an astute critique of academic approaches to popular culture in general, but the problems he raises are exacerbated when the "'typical' or 'average' viewer" against whom critics construct their professional identities occupies an already subordinate cultural position. "Queer visuality" thus comes to occupy a fraught relationship to popular culture and its criticism more generally, which unremember their own sources in visual pleasure and deny "the possibility that scholars might participate with other viewers to imagine or create pleasurably subversive or empowering interpretations of visual culture" (Reed, "Pleasure Manifesto").

Audiences consistently perform the gap between their reactions to *Will and Grace* and critical assumptions about those reactions, a gap that reveals a good deal about the interactions of humor, stereotype, and identification in shaping queer memory. Schiappa cites one critic who, despite "stacking the deck" with clips to prove that *Will and Grace*'s "consistent use of feminine appellations perpetuates the stereotype of the feminized homosexual," found the focus groups responding to these clips saw something else entirely: "Participants noted that such speech-acts constitute 'in jokes' that are acceptable among the gay community and argued that some gay men do, in fact, talk in such ways with each other. Indeed, some . . . gay participants praised such moments as evidence that the show was 'reaching out' to the gay community" (*Beyond Representational Correctness*, 75–76). Another sociological study premised on the idea that viewers laughed at Jack ("that Jack would be seen as 'a fatuous fool and the most frequent butt of humor'") found, instead, that viewers were laughing *with* him ("Jack was seen more as a 'trickster' character").[13] In fact, studies by Schiappa and others of overwhelmingly straight audiences suggest that watching *Will and Grace* decreases homophobic prejudice, especially for people with no other significant exposure to gay culture.

Participants in these studies might well identify with Jack's insouciant response when he finds his "man-tan reunion" has become a play date for suburban gay couples with children. Blissfully oblivious to all the sex-negative, club-negative, camp-negative impulses at work in and on gay culture, Jack pauses, looks around, then says archly, "I'm not really getting the *theme* of this party." Jack's happily wholehearted identification, through his memory of past parties, with the clichés of gay culture — disco music, Broadway musicals, fashion trends — sustains his unwavering confidence in his own sex-positive, camp-positive sensibility. Taking seriously viewers' identifications with Jack shifts our analysis from claims about a meaning somehow inherent in *Will and Grace* to explore a strategy of interpretation — akin to what Eve Sedgwick has called reparative reading — that, like Jack, finds (or creates) pleasure and subcultural identification enabled by subcultural references in the form of memory narratives.[14] Our observations of Web-site chatrooms devoted to *Will and Grace* during the 2000–2001 season confirmed what the focus groups discussed by Schiappa suggest: that viewers — especially young viewers — experienced its campy circulation of memory traces in the form of gay cultural allusions not as a documentary insight into the lives of gay Manhattanites but as an evocation of the pleasures of gay subculture.[15] Not "Just Jack" individually, but *Will and Grace* aroused strong identification with gay subculture among a wide range of viewers, many of whom were not, like the shows' characters, thirtysomething, urban, or gay, but who felt invited by the show to revel in the rich resources of gay memory in ways that enabled the full queer variety of their own manifestations of antagonism toward heteronormativity.

There's Something about Memory

It is not just, or even primarily, the specifics of gay memory that animate *Will and Grace* and seem to constitute viewers' attraction to the show. Rather, it is the way that memory is shown to structure collectivity first through the pleasurable rehearsal of a canon of subcultural references and second through the revision of personal memory narratives (re-valuing that same-sex crush in the first grade, for instance, while down-playing heteronormative participation in a high school prom) in order to reposition oneself in a new community. The now famous two pairs of characters on *Will and Grace*—Will and Grace on one hand, Jack and Karen on the other—represent (among other things) pleasurable or self-denying attitudes toward such memories and, because of that, toward sexuality, self-worth, and community. Viewers' identifications with the characters in this sitcom respond directly to these different dynamics.

Jack, as everyone knows, is the most stereotypically gay character. That is, he most exemplifies gay cultural codes, many of which he enacts through rehearsals of gay memory to create sexual and social bonds with other gay men. In a paradigmatic scene from the second season, when Jack and another man, after eying each other in a store, start to speak, they per-form an updated version of the lyrics from the 1958 movie musical *Gigi,* adapted to express a series of sexual memories ("We met in Soho. / It was the Village. / Gay Pride? / Wigstock. / Ah yes, I remember it well. / In a cage? / On a box. / Vodka neat? / On the rocks. / Ah yes, I remember it well.").[16] Here memory—of both gay cruising habits and of midcentury movie musicals—allows Jack to connect with another gay man and to affirm his sexuality in a way that merges gay eroticism with camp knowl-edge of movies like *Gigi,* cultural geography, and community events, such as Gay Pride and Wigstock. Such quick rehearsals of gay references typified *Will and Grace* so much that when, by the fourth season—in an episode that had the distinction of gaining the largest audience of any episode in the eight years of the show's run[17]—Matt Damon guest-starred as a straight man pretending to be gay so he could join the Gay Men's Chorus European tour, his performance of gayness consisted of parrying cultural references with Jack. Irritated when Damon's character, Owen, interrupts his solo, Jack snaps, "Uh, excuse me. As Aretha said to Gloria, Celine, Shania, and Mariah during Divas Live: 'Are you trippin'? No one inter-rupts the Queen of Soul, bitch. OK?'" only to have Owen snap right back, "Well, I believe she also said, 'Hey, Cuba, Canada, Cowgirl, Crazy, get out of my light and away from my snacks, bitch.'" It is only when Jack catches Owen eying a pretty girl that he starts to suspect that Owen is not gay.

In the end, asserting "a policy of tolerance—we used to have a policy of openness, but that got too many giggles"—the director welcomes the handsome outed-as-straight Owen into the Gay Men's Chorus, leaving Jack to assert, as a feeble last claim not to gayness but to "my dignity," "Yeah? Well, *I* still get to sleep with men."[18]

Displacing medico/scientific definitions of sexual identity based on sex acts with a cultural orientation rooted in memory and citation, *Will and Grace* distinguished itself sharply from other sitcoms, which perpetually reinscribe the dominance of a normative audience by laboriously setting up punch lines that involve subcultural references. Especially when Jack is on screen, *Will and Grace* offers television audiences the unprecedented spectacle of gay subcultural interaction depicted as a practice of shared pleasure for those involved and deployed to include viewers who take their own pleasure in recognizing (which is to say remembering) the sexual scenarios and camp allusions.[19] *Will and Grace* affirms gay memory as a viable basis for belonging, one available even to men who have sex with women but who, like Owen, "love to sing choral music. It makes me feel like I'm [faltering pause] being gently chucked under the chin by God," as Owen reverently puts it. In short, what the privileging of gay memory in *Will and Grace* precludes is not heterosexuality but heteronormativity. And that's quite an accomplishment for a top-ten rated television show.

As virtually every commentary on *Will and Grace* notices, Jack's campy extravagance is counterbalanced by Will Truman. James R. Keller explains the contrast in terms of the characters' names. "The name 'Will' signifies resolution," while his surname "suggests that Will is a 'real man.'" In contrast, the name "Jack" is "a common appellation for a trickster or joker" and has strong sexual connotations, while "'McFarland' suggests both literal and figurative outlandishness" (*Queer (Un)Friendly Film,* 124). True men, possessed of determined will, are apparently less appealing than far-out and eroticized tricksters, as suggested by a survey of college students' favorite character on the show. The only clear loser in the competition was Will (Cooper in Schiappa, *Beyond Representational Correctness,* 78). Similarly, in the NBC chatroom devoted to the show, discussion threads like "*Will & Grace* or Jack & Karen?" and "Who's funnier Will and Grace or Jack and Karen" overwhelmingly elicited responses favoring Jack and Karen (typical among them, "I have been calling it [the show] Jack & Karen for a long time now"). No one favored Will and Grace, and another thread began, "Do you think the reason everyone loves Jack so much is because he is stereotypically gay and Will acts like he's straight?"[20] The affirmative answer seems to be implied by the question itself. Stereotypes, for these viewers, are not turnoffs but imply a cultural literacy and self-acknowledgment that make Jack, not Will, viewers' gay favorite.

Will's contrast with Jack includes his more ambivalent relationship to memory and consequently to gay cultural codes. Except — importantly — under Jack's influence, Will lacks Jack's enthusiasm for the memories attached to camp or cruising, and his own memory narratives regularly rehearse experiences of humiliation and shame: breakups, missed opportunities, childhood embarrassments. Will's is typically the conservative voice, criticizing Jack for his campy deployments of gay codes and for his unembarrassed enjoyment of his sexuality. As a result, unlike Jack, who often mentions friends in what seems an extended gay network, Will is oddly and unhappily isolated, locked into a heterosexual-seeming relationship with Grace (in the show's first episode, they pretend to be newlyweds).

When Will does use memory to make a "love connection," the results don't pay off for him as they do for Jack. Take, for example, the episode in which Jack, working as a Banana Republic salesman, is smitten with Matthew, a handsome shopper.[21] Sensing that Matthew is a "smarty," Jack convinces Will to hide in a dressing room and feed him dialogue through his store headset. Will proffers references that are both straight (John Updike's *Rabbit Run*, for example, which Jack, John Waters–like, turns into "Rabid Nun") and high cultural (shopping for art at the Spielman Gallery). Although the ruse is quickly discovered, and Will and Matthew meet and become a couple, the elite and nongay quality of their memories grounds their relationship in dominant cultural values that quickly become its undoing: a few episodes later they break up when Matthew refuses to challenge his boss's homophobia and acknowledge Will as his lover. By comparison, Jack's carefree display of affection with his latest boyfriend unwittingly "outs" the homophobic boss's son to his dad.[22] In the relationship between Will and Jack, Jack's sexual pleasure and pride repeatedly comprise the trace memory that keeps Will from settling for an elite cultural belonging purchased through shame and disguise.

Not only within the plot of these episodes, but also in relation to the show's audience, Will's rejection of Jack's uninhibited homoeroticism and campy range of reference frustrates ambitions toward community. As numerous chatroom commentators complained, we never see Will and Matthew share an intimate moment.[23] The self-contained nature of their relationship seems to echo the self-contained quality of the memory references on which it is founded. Will and Matthew's initial connection comically exaggerates the mainstream's fixation on individualism: the same individual salesperson at one private gallery tried to sell the same unique work of art to each of them — a memory no one else can share. Where the audience is distanced by Will's range of reference, however, Jack's allusions include us in a community that succeeds in reproducing collective pleasure. Throughout the scene in which Will and Matthew meet through Jack's headset, Jack continually intrudes collective queer memory into their conversation (finding that Matthew works on television, Jack, thinking immediately of the concurrent show, *Buffy, the Vampire Slayer,* exclaims, "Oh my god. I love *Buffy. Buffy* is my life. . . . I'm so into Willow being a lez. Did you have anything to do with that?"). Because he counters their more serious pretensions, Jack, as always, is reproved by Will (and now Matthew) as childish and uncontrolled. Jack seems to speak for the viewing audience, however, when, tired of being excluded by Will and Matthew, he interrupts their conversation with a petulant, "Hey, can we talk about something *I'm* interested in?" Queer viewers might ask much the same thing.

But although Jack is the gayest character, Will is not not-gay. One of the great attractions of *Will and Grace* is its recognition of a range of positions within gay identity.[24] Will often stands up for "gay pride" against straight and potentially homophobic audiences: he organizes a sensitivity training for police officers, insists that his closeted lover acknowledge his sexuality, and is himself vocally "out" in the workplace. Significantly, Will's memory narrative of his sexual identity, staged in the flashback-heavy Thanksgiving 2000 special, credits Jack with pulling him out of the closet. In sharp distinction with the de-generational unremembering that encourages temporal divisions between camp and cruising on the one hand and mainstream politics on the other, the former is presented by *Will and Grace* as a deep history — a collective memory — that enables and remains allied with the more mainstream politics represented by Will.

In the pilot and first few episodes of *Will and Grace,* Will's friendship with Jack was balanced by Grace's relationship with her socialite secretary, Karen. As the sidekicks of the title characters, Karen and Jack did not share the same scenes. Grace, like Will, manifests a difficult relationship to memory, marked by embarrassment and shame (an episode in which guilt motivates Grace's return to Schenectady to apologize to a grade-school classmate whose malicious nickname she initiated, only to be called a "bitch" in front of a funeral parlor full of strangers, is typical).[25] Even the bond between Will and Grace is founded on a shared memory of humiliation occasioned by their failure to achieve normative heterosexuality through sex or marriage. This is the theme of the hour-long 2000 Thanksgiving special, which rehearses their dysfunction in twinned plots — "the story I like to call 'When Mary Met Sally,'" quips Jack — set simultaneously in the past and the present (this structural assertion of the formative relevance of memory is reinforced by the plot, in which these memories are recalled in order to explain to a woman they meet in a bar why her relationship with her obviously gay boyfriend is failing). Not coincidentally, Grace is, like Will, socially awkward and sexually anxious (Karen calls her "Prudence McPrude, Mayoress of Prudie Town").[26] Nevertheless, Grace, also like Will, is capable of fierce loyalty to her gay friends and of an imaginative relation to her own sexuality. If Will's pride relies on his memories of Jack's campy influence, Grace's relies on her memories of Will's steadfast friendship: memory thus fosters bonds not only across differences within the gay community but across supposed divides of gay and straight, male and female.

This passing of memory across boundaries of gender and sexuality is clearest in the character of Karen, nominally a straight woman, who matches Jack's pleasure in eroticism and his repertoire of camp references. Karen's cheerful failure to sustain any conventional social role associated with subordinate femininity — caring wife, nurturing mother, helpful secretary — is linked to Jack's status as the happy homosexual in her response when he asks why she never makes coffee in the office: "For the same reason you don't have a wife and three kids: that's the way god wants it."[27] While Grace is getting called a bitch in Schenectady, Karen tells Jack fondly, "You're simple, you're shallow, and you're a common whore: that's why we're soul mates." And when they argue, Karen is equally equipped from the arsenal of camp knowledge, suddenly quoting *Gypsy,* for instance, as she spits at Jack: "You ain't gettin' eighty-eight cents from me, Rose!"[28] (In a riposte several episodes later into their quarrel, Jack invokes *The Wizard of Oz* to instruct Karen, "Now be gone before someone drops a house on you!")[29] Despite her always-offscreen husband and children, Karen's participation in gay cultural memory "queers" her in ways that become occasionally explicit: when Jack first hears about the man-tan reunion, he tells Grace she can't come because it's "gay guys only," then murmurs to Will, "Remind me to invite Karen."[30] This remark recognizes Karen's character as a hilariously exaggerated projection onto an urban matron of stereotypes of gayness as a self-centered combination of ruthless materialism and devastating wit. "We think she's the gayest thing on television," according to one of the show's creators, contrasting Karen to Jack who "is more wide-eyed, which to me is less campy."[31]

In a television genre that claimed documentary veracity, this attribution of gay stereotypes to middle-aged femininity might seem just one more tediously offensive reminder of the links between homophobia and misogyny; the humiliation of actress Sharon Gless as the progay mom in Showtime's *Queer as Folk* is just one example.[32] In the stylized structure of the sitcom, however, the over-the-top projection of Karen as a best friend for Jack can be enjoyed as a campy inversion of a genre of mainstream films (the 1997 blockbuster *My Best Friend's Wedding* and the derivative *The Next Best Thing*), which projected gay characters (played in both cases by Rupert Everett) solely as handsome and attentive best friends for straight women but with no lives — certainly no gay plots — of their own. This tried-and-true dynamic was the original premise of *Will and Grace*. With the show's success, however, came its confidence to engage directly the common but little-discussed phenomenon of heterosexual women who share enthusiastically in queer cultural codes, while — in a related development — the Jack–Karen relationship grew at least as important as the Will–Grace duo.[33] These shifts coincided, in *Will and Grace*'s second season, with several jabs at the movie precedent: jokes on Grace's insistence that she looks like Julia Roberts, the star of *My Best Friend's Wedding* (Karen responds, "The only thing you two have in common is horse teeth and bad taste in men"),[34] an episode titled "My Best Friend's Tush," and, most noticeably, the ongoing plot in which Karen arranges Jack's marriage of convenience to her maid, mocking the heterosexual romantic conventions of the films from which the show derived.

For all of the four main characters in *Will and Grace*, the ability to deploy and revise stereotypes and to make community across identities often conceived as antagonistic is enabled by memory: personal memories of the characters' shared histories and, more important, cultural memories shared by a community of viewers. Insisting that gay subcultural memory can create community across differences of sexual politics, gender, or class, *Will and Grace* exemplifies the potential of gay memory both to cohere and to transform — to "queer" — contemporary notions of identity.

"Jack Has Originality": Subversive Sensibility and Subcultural Belonging

Our own pleasure in *Will and Grace* derives in part from the scarcity of popular representations of gay memory. The hunger for such representations is often belittled in mainstream television commentary, but one sign of the dominant culture's privilege is its failure to recognize its own rehearsals of collective memory for what they are. People invested in normative identities (whiteness, maleness, heterosexuality) that are continually reinforced by mainstream media as the makings of unique individuality can afford to ignore the collective aspect of those memories. To be a privileged citizen is to imagine oneself an autonomous individual, although — or because — that "individuality" looks a lot like everyone else's.

For those marginalized from mainstream culture, however, memories on which to ground alternative social identities must be more self-consciously recognized, cultivated, and shared. This self-consciousness, performed in relation to mass culture, is the basic component of camp, which Sontag describes as a "way of seeing the world as an aesthetic phenomenon" ("Notes on Camp," 279). The force of the "aesthetic" in Sontag's analysis is emphasized in her description of "taste": "To patronize the faculty of taste is to patronize oneself. For taste governs every free — as opposed to rote — human response" (278). For Sontag, taste is manifest not simply in preferences for certain kinds of art or people; "there is taste in acts, taste in morality. Intelligence, as well, is really a kind of taste: taste in ideas" (278). To respond campily, therefore, is to abjure the "rote" responses privileged by the dominant culture as individualism in favor of "a mode of enjoyment, of appreciation" (293) that "turns its back on the good–bad axis of ordinary aesthetic judgment. . . . It doesn't argue the good is bad, or the bad is good. What it does is to offer for art (and life) a different — a supplementary — set of standards" (288).

As a disruptive mode of interpretation that inverts authoritative claims to meaning and hierarchies of value, camp is notoriously hard to define, except by example. We find camp's power exemplified in the *Will and Grace* episode "I Never Promised You an Olive Garden" (the title is itself a campy memory reference to Lynn Anderson's 1970 hit, "I Never Promised You a Rose Garden"). In this episode, Karen goads Jack into overcoming his traumatic memories of grade-school bullies so that he will accompany her to a principal's conference at her stepchildren's posh academy. There Jack encounters young John, who is being bullied just as Jack was as a child. Identifying with John, Jack thwarts the bullies first by camping it up (he grabs Karen's purse and condemns physical aggression from a fashion standpoint: "This macho bully schoolyard crap is *so* 1983 I could vomit. Now scram!"), then by sharing gay cultural codes with John (showing him how to perform "Just John" with Jack's signature "jazz hands"). Here the camp frivolity of fashion, femininity, and song-and-dance trumps the thudding viciousness of the normative hands down — or, rather, up, and with a snap. Memory is crucial to this episode, as Jack inducts John into a camp sensibility that, shared with others, becomes subcultural belonging. Jack teaches John how to be himself, a self that is both Jack and John. Here queer memories are rescued from the trauma of isolated individualism (being alone, being beaten up) and transformed into a shared identity that empowers and delights both participants. "Thanks for your help," John says. "Same here," Jack replies.[35]

The differences between mainstream and camp deployments of memory, and the different kinds of subjectivity they produce, are explicitly at issue in "My Best Friend's Tush." In this episode, Jack invents a cushion for mass-transit riders called "the Subway Tush" (his focus is on a collective experience of public pleasure outside the mainstream American identification with the individualism of the automobile and the privacy of bodily sensation). When Will's refusal to fund Jack's scheme is overcome by Grace (typically, using a heterosexualizing plot that infantilizes Jack, she pleads to Will, "I work all day. You work all day. He comes home at 3:00 to an empty house. I worry about him."), Will arranges a meeting with potential investors. Although Jack makes Will promise to talk to the investors on his behalf, once they assemble, Jack can't resist bursting into song ("Hey *mon frère* / If your *derrière* / Needs a little cush . . ."). The investors are sold by Jack's campy performance but want the straight-laced Will out of the venture because he thinks "too small." To spare Will's feelings, Jack lies about the investors' motives, but when Will asserts they are backing out because "you turned a meeting with my colleagues into Circus-O-Gay," Jack tells the truth, profoundly upsetting Will's sense of himself as the acceptable face of homosexuality. Will's funk lasts until Grace reveals that Jack is quitting the venture out of loyalty to Will. When Will interrupts the meeting where Jack plans to dismiss his investors, he bursts in with a speech promoting Jack ("Jack has . . . passion, he has vision, and most of all, Jack has originality. There is not an idea in this man's head that is not fresh, unique"), only to learn that the deal has foundered because Jack stole the idea for the Subway Tush from "an ex-lover of Swedish extraction."

In this plot, Jack and Will express very different notions of originality and what it implies for individuality and community. For Will, original-ity — unique individual self-possession — is the basis of vision and passion. Jack, however, has knowingly both taken the idea for the Subway Tush from Bjorn and derived his campy promotional shtick from commercial jingles. Jack's undeniable passion and vision do not, as Will claims, derive from his originality but from his sly powers of citation. In episode after episode, Jack's erotic and social repertoire recycles mass-media memo-ries, passing them through his camp sensibility — montage and medley are his fortes — for the pleasure of his friends and of television audiences. If Jack's performances are who he is (his cabaret act is called "Just Jack!"), then it is notably untrue that "Jack has originality." Jack's identity — and his passions — are clearly constructed through his sharing of gay subcul-tural bonds (including his sexual relationship with Bjorn). Will, in his rush for mainstream acceptance, mislabels these acts as "originality," fail-ing to value them — at least for this audience of suits — as moments of collectively recycled and mass-mediated queer memory.[36]

For some critics, Will's pandering to potential investors might be para-digmatic of what is wrong with *Will and Grace*. Critiques of mass media for selling out gay culture through a combination of niche marketing for gay audiences and assimilationist depictions of gay men are not wrong, just incomplete.[37] The evolution of gay identity in tandem with emerging forms of commercial entertainment suggests a symbiotic relationship between the two as mass-media niche marketing helps to create what it presumes: a community that shares a set of references and attitudes.[38] Primary among those attitudes in the case of gay identity is camp, a practice of pleasure first nurtured and taught in niche commercial spaces (primarily bars and theaters) and later in niche commercial publications — including some academic venues — where critics lovingly explicated the camp subtexts of mass-marketed entertainments (primarily films and novels).[39] As a strategy for the useful misreading of popular culture, camp helps to repair the mass media's corrosive effects on gay subculture, cultivating an actively ironic viewership in place of the gullible passivity presumed of audiences by these media's harsher critics.

Will and Grace's depiction of camp strategies circulating within an explicitly gay context opens a new commercialized venue for the cultivation of gay memory, and the Subway Tush investors' fascination with Jack's campy advertising jingle seems self-consciously to parallel the campy Old Navy ads (featuring Megan Mullally, the actress who plays Karen) that punctuated the original airings of the show. Though this is a shift more in scale than in kind from earlier commercial circulations of camp, the new scale does, significantly, widen the interpretive community for gay memory that is synergistically presumed and created by any performance of camp. Undoubtedly, some of the intensity and subversiveness of gay subcultural identification is traded for wider relevance, a move that echoes the broader cultural shift from relatively separatist and small "gay" and "lesbian" communities to broader but vaguer "queer" counterpublics. Jack's performances of camp deploy a repertoire of codes available to anyone — male or female, gay or straight — with access to the same forms of mass media. *Will and Grace* allows the women characters to pick up on Jack's strategy of using media references to disrupt conventional logics of conversation and plot. Karen's cultural references are perfectly in sync with Jack's, but even the more normative Grace has her moments: in a scene where Will tries to distance Grace by hissing bitterly, "You might as well be my wife," Grace deflects the insult by pretending to mishear him, responding incredulously, "Marcus Welby's my wife?" To camp on mass culture may make one less "original," less possessed of the unique individualism signaled by one's embodiment of a stable, autonomous "identity." But to dismiss mass entertainment for "selling out" gay culture misses the complex interactions between commercial co-optation and resistant interpretation, autonomous identity and cross-cultural identifications, individualism and the imagined community of viewers. The practices of camp that *Will and Grace* depicts suggest that queers can co-opt mass culture and not just the other way around, allowing through such acts of reparative interpretation the possibilities for collective originality to emerge.

"I Guess Weddings Just Bring Out the Worst in Me"

The challenge that the recycling of queer cultural memory poses to the oxymoron of conventional individuality extends to that corollary of individualism: the perfect couple. What most distinguishes Will and Grace from Jack and Karen may be their differing relationship to the ideal of the all-consuming self-sufficiency of the couple. Will and Grace seem happiest, as evidenced in the failed experiment with Grace moving across the hall, when they are in the same apartment, uninterrupted by visits — usually presented as "intrusions" — by Jack and Karen. What the title characters reinforce, then, is an overdetermined image of the conventional nuclear family: Mom and Dad happily ensconced in their private home, with two unruly interlopers (boy and girl child) who are affectionately indulged, though not treated as equals. This depiction has troubling consequences: it desexualizes Grace and Will (especially Will, whose homosexuality is repeatedly blamed for their failure to find complete fulfillment in each other); it presents queers as developmentally immature (emotional "children" who will grow into a "mature" recognition of the values represented by Will and Grace); and, above all, it validates a way of life cut off from the pleasures brought by broader social formations.

Jack and Karen, in contrast, circulate promiscuously. While we typically see Will and Grace only at home or at work unless brought to another space by Jack and Karen, the latter are often in stores, restaurants, gyms, hotels, schools: all spaces that enable interaction with people — often queer people — who float in and out of the plot, often without names or fully developed characters.[40] These spaces and interactions allow Jack and Karen more fluid and expansive definitions of relationships, community, and identity. Despite — or maybe because of — their outrageous narcissism, which allows them to assume that everyone they encounter shares their sensibility, there is an element of generosity in Jack's and Karen's relationships to the broader social world that is absent in Will and Grace's tightly controlled, hermetic environment. Jack's and Karen's disruptions of the couple-centric dynamic is a crucial part of the appeal of *Will and Grace,* allowing the show to take its place with *Friends* (another hit sitcom that, to judge from chatroom discussions and network marketing strategies, shares a significant component of its audience of young adults with *Will and Grace*) as a forum in which the contradictory dynamics of couple and community are negotiated for viewers at the stage in life when mainstream norms demand the prioritization of "the couple" and marriage over friendship networks created in school.

These issues are explicitly at play in an episode titled "Coffee and Commitment," which involves the four regulars in the commitment ceremony of Joe and Larry (the former fast-life gay couple turned suburban dads already mentioned in connection with the failed man-tan reunion). "I love weddings," is Grace's immediate couple-centric response. "Well, it's not strictly a wedding; it's a same-sex civil union, which affords many of the same rights as a marriage," responds Will, articulating his legalistic grasp on the limitations of the dominant culture's acceptance of gay couples as affirming reflections of heteronormative values. Will and Grace's reflection of the usual range of liberal debate on this issue is interrupted by Jack in a caffeine-induced delirium, announcing, "Did you see that? I almost did the half nelson. I almost bruised my delicates, my delicates, my domo arigato Mr. Tomatoes. Huge news! I have met — Are you ready for this? Mr. Right. Well, Mr. Right-Now, anyway. Ba-da-bum. Good night, folks, I'm here all week. Jack 2000!" Conventional coupledom doesn't stand a chance in the face of this promiscuous collapse of boundaries not only between couples but between languages, between denotation and euphemism, between authentic expressions of individual emotions and cultural clichés, between personal conversation and public performance.

The episode goes on to juxtapose the mock-hetero gay couple with the addictions of Jack (to caffeine) and Karen (to booze and pills), as Will and Grace angrily debate their own emotional and financial commitment to one another. This pairing of plots reflects the situation of sexual minorities today, caught between stereotyped ideals of conventional coupling and equally stereotyped diagnoses of gay culture as a morass of disease and addiction. The episode's yoking of "commitment" and "addiction" suggests that one can end up addicted to the conventional rituals of the exclusive couple (in the final scene, Grace says of the wedding cake she is addictively gobbling, "It's got nine layers of chocolate and a Snickers bar in the middle. I may move into it"). This addiction, the episode suggests, has particularly bad effects on gay men, who end up "picking up the bill" (Will is angry throughout the episode about Grace's assumption that he will pay for the wedding present and all their joint ventures). More figuratively, gay men pick up the bill for conventional coupledom by submitting themselves to conventional gender roles (Larry and Bob wonder which is the bride), social isolation (no more man-tan parties in the Hamptons for this happy couple; in a later episode, Larry and Bob cancel a trip to Morocco with Will, unwilling to leave their daughter Hannah behind), and a sense of shame about alternative erotic or romantic arrangements. As Will tells Grace, "I guess weddings just bring out the worst in me."

Representing an alternative — and today often vilified — gay legacy, Jack and Karen, the explicitly "addicted" characters, end up supplying each other with a form of companionship and support that is harder to ritualize and hence to name (they decide to get over the DTs by "touching each other inappropriately"), but no less trustworthy for that. And *their* addictions — to pleasure in its myriad forms — lead not to exclusion and shame but to inclusion (Jack flirts with a man who offers him a cigarette; Karen finds booze by seeking out the inevitable "sad sister," shamed by her single status at the marriage of her gay brother). If addiction to conventional coupledom brings out the worst in Will and Grace, addictions to pleasure — reinforced through the expansive communities built through shared memory and circulated cultural codes — bring out the best in Jack and Karen. This episode suggests that the collective identities built through gay memory model at least one alternative to gay (or even, in the case of Will and Grace, queer) marriage and the exclusive couple.

The History of the Queer Future

Out of our memories come our futures. Not only what we remember but *how* we remember — with pleasure or pain, generosity or anxiety — shapes the futures we will enjoy (or endure) as communities or as individuals. This is the theme of the episode "There But for the Grace of Grace," in

which Will and Grace make a pilgrimage to visit a beloved college professor, Joseph Dudley. They find him disillusioned and embittered, locked in a
battle of resentments with his longtime companion, Sharon. Watching the
two snipe at one another, Will and Grace recognize aspects of their own
relationship. Grace exclaims to Will, "Them. They're us," adding, "When
he put down the bottle of Correctol by her lamb chop, she said 'Ew.' I say
'Ew.' Will, she is exactly who I'm going to be." This return to the past gives
Grace a vision of her future, a vision she uses to change the course of
her history. When Grace tells Sharon that she terminated an engagement
after Will disapproved of the man, Sharon confronts Grace with, "Because
god forbid there should be any other man in your life besides Will." Sharon
recognizes that her relationship with Joseph has prevented both of them
from exploring the potential range of their pleasures, locking them into a
life of frustrated resentment. Will and Grace learn their lesson from this
trip down memory lane: a few episodes later, Will encourages Grace to
pursue a relationship with her new romantic interest and in the process
meets a man he has admired bashfully from afar.

Of course, Grace's immediate history always held a potentially "queer"
future. Her own mother, Bobbi (played by Debbie Reynolds), is never
depicted with her husband; instead, we see her with her effeminate ac-
companist with whom she performs a camp repertoire of show tunes and
disco hits. Although Grace asserts her difference from her mother, they
both share a love of gay men and the culture they produce (Bobbi asks
Grace, "What do the boys make out to these days? Is it still Judy?").[41]
Grace's past, rightly remembered, thus offers her another means of escape from Sharon's frustrations into the pleasures and possibilities of a
queer future.

Grace, in a later episode, offers Will a similar view into his queer future
when she gives him a visit to the clairvoyant, Psychic Sue, as a birthday
gift. Sue predicts that Will will be contacted by a "strawberry blonde" with
whom he once had a relationship and to whom he never got a chance to say
good-bye. When she identifies this blonde as a "she," Will dismisses Sue's
predictions as heterosexist smoke and mirrors, only to return home to find
a package from his mother containing the collar of his beloved childhood
pet, a strawberry blonde dog that died while Will was away at college. Sue
has plunged Will back into his past, and his memory, like virtually all his

memories, is at best bittersweet, associating affection with loss and disappointment. It is Grace who queers Will's memory: when he takes out the dog collar and announces it belonged to "Ginger," Grace asks, "That drag queen you and Jack hung out with last summer?" Will's memory takes him to his nuclear family, a site, as always for him, of pain. Grace's comment, however, suggests a competing history: not of pain but of pleasure, not of heterosexuality but of queer gender-bending, not of childhood innocence but of adult sexual play. Above all, the memory Grace evokes is collective: involving not just Jack but also someone with at best a contingent relation to Will's life (someone he "hung out with" for a summer) but who has nevertheless functioned as a source of queer pleasure, and the pleasure of this memory—for the laughing audience if not for Will—defuses the heavy sentimentality of Will's maudlin family memory.

As textual critics like to say, this scene is foreshadowing, for when, now convinced of Sue's psychic acumen, Will returns for a second visit, he wants to know what, romantically, awaits him in his future. Sue reveals to him that he will spend the rest of his life with someone named Jack, a revelation that upsets Will. Much of the episode's humor centers on his hysterical distaste for the idea of sexual union with Jack. Two narratives run side by side here. In one, Will seeks pleasure in a memory rooted in a past dominated by the heterosexual nuclear family (a memory that, we can see even if he cannot, brings him pain). This familial memory, projected into the future, conjures a kind of mirror image: another man exactly like Will to play the missing half of his ideal couple. In contrast, the queer memory—of the drag queen who might have worn a dog collar—takes Will to another future, shared with Jack. That future will be very different from Will's normative ideal: when Jack learns of Sue's prediction, he insists that, in his "marriage" to Will, each must have his own apartment and his own boyfriends. The future with Jack—a future predicated on a "memory" of a summer spent "hanging out" (as opposed to Will's usual mode, "staying in")—busts the conventional couple wide open, suggesting a future founded in pleasure, gender nonconformity, sexual play, and above all, expansive community, not in the sentimental innocence of the exclusive couple.[42]

In all these episodes, *Will and Grace* suggests that memories can function not as signposts toward a future for which we are inevitably fated

(or doomed) but as the materials from which we can construct new relationships to our communities and a new sense of self. Using memory to
create new futures requires several steps, as these episodes demonstrate.
First, queers must learn to identify not according to biological "sameness"
(sons must follow their fathers) but across cultural differences of sexuality,
gender, and lifestyle. While these queered identifications may disrupt the
nuclear family (Will's relationship to his own childhood) and the conventional couple (Will and Grace's sense of themselves as almost-married),
they open up possibilities for new and expansive communities, which
may include biological relations (like Bobbi) or conventional couples (like
Larry and Bob) but are not restricted to them. Our memories take us,·
then, to places and people who, in our past, gave us pleasure (sexual pleasure, perhaps, but also the pleasures of good conversation, new experiences, and fresh perspectives). These people and places are often erased by
conventional sources of memory (albums featuring photos only of weddings, babies, or family gatherings), but their memories are carried by the
traces of mass culture that allowed us to meet them in the first place and
that gave us a shared vocabulary of remembrance. These cultural sources
carry the memories of collective pleasure, whether in Bobbi's rendition of
the disco hit "Gloria," in Karen's citations of *Gypsy,* or Grace's reference to
drag, all of which recalls a history of gender nonconformity and campy
defiance. Out of these memories, *Will and Grace* forms a new community
and invites us, if we are willing to let the memories be ours, to share its
pleasures.

Thanks for the Memories

Debates over gay memory and identity can make us feel that we must
choose sides. What'll it be: memory or amnesia, community or couples,
subculture or assimilation? One of the pleasures of *Will and Grace* is its
use of humor to stage an optimistic hope for resolution of debilitating debates within the gay community between the positions Michael Warner
describes as "the dignified homosexual" and the "queer who flaunts his
sex and his faggotry, making the dignified homosexual's stigma all the
more justifiable in the eyes of straights" (*The Trouble with Normal,* 32). In
place of this antagonistic scenario, *Will and Grace* repeatedly shows Jack

pulling Will from his isolation, encouraging him into rehearsals of gay memory. Together they recall sexual exploits and perform apparently spontaneous yet carefully choreographed campy duets that suggest Will's unacknowledged store of gay memory. In return, Will protects Jack, providing him the emotional and financial support that allows him to pursue his more transgressive behaviors. This rapprochement between forms of gay identity that are often presented as antagonistic is crucial to the show's appeal, defusing a disabling sense of incoherence not only among different kinds of gay men but within individuals defining their own sexual identity. "I am totally like Will, but I have a flouncing Jack inside of me waiting to come out and meet people," reads one posting in a chatroom devoted to the show.[43]

Another aspect of *Will and Grace*'s appeal is its delight in exploring the bonds between certain forms of gay male and straight female identity, and by extension the validation it offers for relationships between gay men and straight women, reversing the pejorative view of both parties implied in the common epithet "fag hag."[44] The affirmation *Will and Grace* offers a queer community of gay men and their straight women friends does not depend primarily on plot, however. Other television shows have presented supposedly gay characters in friendship plots without gaining the powerful allegiance of gay viewers (the short-lived sitcom *Normal, Ohio*, which ran during *Will and Grace*'s third season, for example). What *Will and Grace* offers beyond demographic representation is a range of relationships to gay memory and identity, and most important, the continual, delighted, and delightful engagement of the audience in the dynamics of queer identity formation through a sensibility founded in memory. As campy references to the gay past and contemporary queer mores whiz past, we recognize, we recall, we repeat these remarks in ways that value not only the specific allusions to elements of gay history but the related strategies of campy interpretation and performance that lie at the heart of gay cultural memory.

Will and Grace's role in producing identifications with gay memories through the circulation of cultural references is reflected in many remarks posted in chatrooms performed to the show, where the recognition–recall–repeat dynamic is performed again and again. The question "Are any guys/girls in a 'Will and Grace' friendship??" elicited such responses as:

My best friend and I are soooooooo Will and Grace.

It's scary sometimes because a lot of the things that happen on the show resemble things that have happened to us. . . . Sometimes we all get together and have Will and Grace night at someone's house.

My best friends ARE most definitely Will and Grace, no doubt about it. We love the show and although we can't always be together to watch it, we always analyze it soon after. And we are always quoting the show.

My best friend and I watch the show together every week and more and more I see W&G jokes popping into our everyday conversations! We continue to frighten people wherever we go.[45]

This dynamic is especially clear in a posting from "Eddie T.," who writes: "I'm really tuning in to Jack & Karen each week. Sean & Megan [Sean Hayes and Megan Mullally, who play Jack and Karen] make the world seem a little safer for those of us who are still inventing ourselves, but in spite of the reception we get, are not unpleased with where we've gotten so far—any day now we're gonna find that pony."[46] Eddie recognizes that viewers' identifications are not necessarily with a simple demographic category (I'm a gay man, so I identify with a gay character) but with the process of "inventing" identity as part of a social relationship forged from cultural citation and memory, no less important for having been derived from mass media (he concludes his posting by invoking one of Karen's lines from the show). The importance of such references is also registered in queries motivated by viewers' desire to expand their range of camp references and attitudes. "I really wanna know the name of the song Will and Jack sang to the baby," opened one thread. About Karen, female posters confess, "At times I wish that I had the nerve to say what she says to people who tick me off! My fav line: 'Love ya like a cold sore!'" and "Karen is the woman I want to be! . . . To be able to completely overlook all my MANY flaws and just roast everyone I see. That takes guts and quite a bit of confidence."[47]

We do not claim that the world will change because one more person can identify Patti LaBelle's 1974 "Lady Marmalade" or somebody somewhere learns to stand up for herself with a quick and campy put-down. Nor is *Will and Grace* adequate to the needs of queer representation. No television show could be, of course, and the limitations of class, race, geographical setting, and other particulars beg for more sitcoms—and other cultural phenomena—to address a wider demographic range of queer-ness. Even within the demography *Will and Grace* claims as its own, two of the show's shortcomings were always glaringly evident: the absence of lesbians and of explicit gay eroticism.

For a show that was otherwise so good on the dynamics of queer in-clusion, the absence of lesbians is particularly disappointing and seems to reflect long-outdated notions that gay men and lesbians exist in entirely separate cultural spaces (when lesbians are referred to, it's almost always in a put-down by Jack, reinforcing old stereotypes of misogynistic gay men). Several lesbians who are central figures in queer cultural mem-ory—Martina Navratilova, Sandra Bernhard, Ellen DeGeneres—made cameo appearances on the show, yet the lesbian presence in mass media that these figures represent was never mined as part of the queer mem-ory *Will and Grace* built on. By the same token, the enormous contribu-tion of lesbians to queer social and political organizations goes oddly and unhappily unreflected in the community modeled by *Will and Grace*, an absence registered in the lack of self-identified lesbian participants in the show's chatrooms.

The other major shortcoming, which viewers in the chatrooms regu-larly lamented, is *Will and Grace*'s failure to show gay erotic interaction, this in contrast to the way heterosexuals regularly kiss, cuddle, and appear in bed together.[48] In the episode "The Young and the Tactless," for instance, Grace is seduced by a neighbor, Nathan, whom she professes to find re-pulsive until he overcomes her torrent of words with a kiss.[49] By contrast, in the following episode, Will is allowed only a quick peck on the lips with the young video-store clerk he is dating. In a dynamic where gay eroticism can be discussed but never pictured, this trumping of words by the taboo of the visualized deed allows heterosexuality to trump homo-sexuality in the show's hierarchy of pleasures. Significantly, this is the same episode in which certain verbal taboos are broken, with an overt display of homophobia directed at Will and Jack by Karen's mother-in-law. The show's apparent willingness to stage visual heteroeroticism and verbal homophobia but not visual homoeroticism remains a disappoint-ing reflection of mainstream squeamishness.

As *Will and Grace* continued after the third season, moreover, its plot-lines veered increasingly toward the romance plots that are the staple of most sitcoms. This may be explained, in part, by the departure of the original creative team responsible for the show (David Kohan and Max Mutchnick wrote only one episode in the fourth season and then became embroiled in a protracted legal battle with the network, not returning until the final episode of the final season).[50] Mainstream critics welcomed this development: "Now that Grace has got herself a boyfriend, the series has improved beyond all recognition. The astringent wisecracking is still there, but it no longer exists within the hermetically sealed world of gay culture" (Chater, "Viewing Guide"). But then, they never understood the popularity of the show. The TV columnist for that bastion of normativity *USA Today* heralded the end of the show with, "All those insults and pop-culture quips did more than just hinder the development of the characters; they buried them. Eight years later, we still have no idea of who these people are or what they want" (Bianco, "So Who, Exactly, Were Those People?"). Who people are is necessarily distinct, for this reviewer, from "pop-culture quips." Yet it is precisely those cultural references that make a sense of queer belonging that — for the characters as well as the majority of viewers who weigh in on chatrooms — is exactly "what they want."[51] The show played to such desires, although increasingly the longing for belongings *outside* the couple gave way to the pleasures of coupling *in opposition* to broader cultural formations. Like Grace, Will coupled up in a long-term relationship; in a move that seems calculated to emphasize his normativity, his partner was a policeman. These moves put increasing pressure on the characters of Jack and Karen to sustain the show's campy exuberance, a challenge to which they often rose.

When the original creators of the series were brought back for the 2006 series finale, they inherited these plots and attempted to offer the characters resolution. The conclusion, in some ways, reflected the dynamic of the later seasons. Jack and Karen have sustained a relationship so queer it defies categorization: they trade witticisms, lift their shirts and touch tummies, and — in a musical tribute to the importance of memory — sing the old crooner's classic "Unforgettable" to one another. Grace and Will, on the other hand, have drifted apart under the pressure of childrearing and marriage (albeit same-sex marriage in Will's case). Their college-age children are now engaged, and the show threatens to end with the heteronormative marriage Will and Grace would have had if Will had not been gay. At the last minute, however, the plot returns them to a reunion with Jack and Karen in the bar that was the setting for the first episode. Belying critical imperatives to demonstrate growth and maturity by falling into normative affiliations, the show ends with Will's observation, "You know what's funny? We haven't changed a bit." And Grace responds, "It's kinda nice, isn't it?"[52]

We prefer to conclude, however, with the final episode of *Will and Grace*'s 2001 season, which returned to the power and promise of queer memory. In this episode, Jack is set up to believe that he is finally going to meet his father, Joe Black, only to discover that his father died some years ago. When Will tries to comfort Jack, they express their different understandings of memory.

JACK: He'll never teach me to ride a bike or throw a ball or kiss a man. I'm totally alone.

WILL: Jack, what have you really lost here? I mean, it would have been great if you'd gotten to know him, but he wasn't part of your life before, he's not part of your life now. What's really changed?

JACK: But I loved him.

WILL: But you didn't *know* him.

JACK: But I loved him.

WILL: Maybe you loved the *idea* of him.[53]

In contrast to Will's belief that memories must be based on "actual" relations (particularly biological ones), Jack understands that memories are concepts ("ideas") that ground who we are in the present. Telling Will, "He was the source of all my talents," Jack affirms what viewers of *Will and Grace* have already seen: Jack's "talents" arise from an affectionate attachment to self-generated memories, the products of mass media and camp (Jack's notion of filial affection is derived, typically, from a movie; throughout the episode, he sings Barbra Streisand's *Yentl* hit, "Papa Can You Hear Me?") rather than of biological kinship. Out of these memories, Jack develops self-affirmation (noting that his talents are his father's, Jack, in claiming that he "loves" his father, is saying he loves himself) and collective attachment (without his memories, Jack is alone).

More important, having detached his memories from his particular history, Jack allows them to circulate in unpredictable ways. Strikingly, it is Grace's new boyfriend, Nathan, who proves best able to understand Jack's affectionate relationship to memory. Proposing a memorial service where he, Jack, and Will share memories that are necessarily self-generated (none of them knew Joe Black), Nathan makes the following toast:

> We're born, we grow, we live, we die. If we're lucky, we have family and friends who know us and love us. I never knew my dad. But it doesn't matter, because wherever we go and whatever we do, we know that the spirit of the mother and the spirit of the father are alive in each of us, that everything good already exists within ourselves. So, here's to Joe, the father in all of us.

Like Jack, Nathan understands that each of us has a "Joe," a memory we use to bolster our talents and everything else that is best in us. That memory is less register of an actual event or person than a projection of a desire for connection, for kinship, for community. If making such memories a "father" that gives rise to a present-day "family" seems heterosexualizing and patriarchal, the circulation of this memory between Nathan and Jack ensures that fathers can be gay (indeed, in a subplot of the episode, Jack discovers he is the father of a boy, Elliot, conceived from a sperm donation to a lesbian played by Rosie O'Donnell), that families are what we make, not just what we are born into. In short, family functions here as shorthand for community, and the community the show imagines, built from the stuff of queer memory (here conventional notions of family themselves are queered), extends across identities, sexualities, and genders.

Of course, one never can enter fully into a community made with the dead—or, for that matter, with characters on television sitcoms—but there is even something queer about the friction between individual affect and fictive collectivity, echoing what Christopher Nealon describes as an ongoing tension within gay representation between "the unspeakability of desire . . . and group life," as manifest in collective cultural forms (*Foundlings*, 13). While we are not urging an uncritical relation to either mass media or to the queer cultures it enables and shapes, we are asserting the value of taking pleasure in a continually changing and multifaceted gay memory and in the mass media that are its repository. The memories generated by television run the risk, as Lipsitz warns, of making "culture . . . seem like a substitute for politics, a way of posing only imaginary solutions to real problems," or worse, "internalizing the dominant culture's norms and values as necessary and inevitable" (*Time Passages*, 16).

Yet, as Lipsitz recognizes, "Culture can become a rehearsal for politics" and even "a form of politics" (16). At their best, television sitcoms extend the legacy of the popular theater as "a kind of free space of the imagination" where "desire does not have to be justified or explained" (9). But the best of the medium demands the best of its viewers: our willingness to use the pleasurable identifications it arouses to transcend passive consumption and become the embodied practice of community. In so doing, we might see the pleasures produced by mass culture, even the most anonymous of its media, television, as the means to code-making systems of memory- and affect-production that allow the shared discourse of queer community in the present and the future.

4. QUEER THEORY IS BURNING

Sexual Revolution and Traumatic Unremembering

Trauma/Theory

The history of AIDS in the United States and the history of queer theory in the academy overlap almost exactly. Beginning with the publication of Eve Kosofsky Sedgwick's *Between Men* in 1985, the academic purchase of queer theory grew in tandem with the mounting horror caused by the spread of AIDS. Most important for our purposes here, the advent of AIDS and the first wave of queer theory (spanning roughly the decade between 1985 and 1995) both seemed to mark a clear division between the past and its own present.[1] Just as gay life after AIDS became sharply severed from life before the epidemic, queer theory came to seem conceptually discontinuous with critical work inspired by the gay liberation movement (it is difficult to imagine, for example, a seminar in queer theory that prioritized the work of members of the pioneering Gay Academic Union, such as Karla Jay, Jonathan Ned Katz, and Barbara Gittings). The first wave of queer theory, of course, included sophisticated AIDS activists who never forgot the cultures AIDS eclipsed, Douglas Crimp, Cindy Patton, Simon Watney, and Paula Treichler among them.[2] For the most part, however, early queer theorists took little account of AIDS or of previous generations of critics. Accusing those who kept company with the past of naïve essentialism, queer theorists turned a blind eye to the historical conditions of queer theory's own meteoric rise within the academy and the trauma that the unremembering necessary to that rise produced *as* queer critical methodology.

One might speculate that the habits of unremembering that proliferated in the first decade of the epidemic played a role in queer theory's rapid growth within the academy. Just as newly "respectable" gays and lesbians who repudiated the immature self-indulgences of the past became more acceptable within mainstream politics, so the first generation of queer theorists, translating the exuberant challenges to institutions (including universities) put forward by activist groups like the Gay Academic Union (GAU) into abstract forces of subversion (melancholy, self-shattering *jouissance,* the death drive), found themselves enthusiastically welcomed at the curricular table of prestigious universities. As we have suggested, however, the apparent break with the past invoked in calls for unremembering in this era was illusory: not a clean break but an anxious self-policing of (the desire for) memory, making unremembering into a traumatic discipline. Although the first wave of queer theory, we argue in what follows, only seemed to sever its ties with the past, its propensity for unremembering provoked the critical preoccupations of the second generation. Much second-wave queer theory is preoccupied by what Michael Snediker, as quoted in our Introduction, calls the "tropaic gravitation toward negative affect" (*Queer Optimism,* 4), such as rage, shame, and loss; by temporal disorientation and "queer time"; and by the present melancholy that also becomes queerness's disruptive future. These, we argue, are signs of a post-traumatic response to the first wave's own traumatized forgetting not only of AIDS but of the critical work of gays and lesbians living before AIDS. In what follows, our interest lies primarily with those second-wave queer theorists whose first significant work in that field was published after 1995 and who have the most to gain from engaging and reversing their predecessors' unremembering.

To assign post-traumatic symptoms to a critical movement might seem far-fetched, but striking points of comparison link the symptoms of post-traumatic disorder and recent trends in queer theory. Unremembering is typically cited as an *effect* of trauma for survivors, but forgetting might just as plausibly *cause,* as well as result from, trauma. In this logic, unremembering produces a post-traumatic disorder readable both through the occlusion of the past (the forgetting of prior acts of traumatic unremembering) and through four secondary symptoms frequently seen in those suffering post-traumatically. First, a history of abuse that is unremembered (here the forgotten unremembering) becomes ritual self-abuse, often manifest in feelings of inner absence or lack. This translation of historically specific abuse into internalized lack requires a high degree of abstraction (in that "lack" requires neither specific causes nor effects). Second, the positive aspects of a traumatized past (what can be half-remembered around the edges of lack) are recast as futural aspirations (what one wants when one "works through" trauma). This might lead to either a romanticizing of futurity or its vilification as the time of unachievable reparation. Third, unable to locate the cause of trauma, those suffering post-traumatically often experience free-floating rage, sadness, and shame, divorced from their historical object and reattached to the sufferer's own incapacity to achieve happiness, an inability often blamed on the desire for human connection itself. Finally, the traumatized experience a strong sense of time gone awry, of living in the past and the present simultaneously, the past seeming to be more in front of one, temporally, than behind, while the future takes on the displaced form of the past.[3]

This list of symptoms, with the word "sexuality" substituted for "trauma," might stand as a catalog of second-wave queer theory's critical preoccupations and strategies. First, the focus on melancholy, usually removed from any but a generalized oedipal cause, provides the abstracted "lack" that turns historically specific traumas into self-generating melancholy. Historically specific loss — of those who died from AIDS, of the lost social worlds many of them made, of memories of those losses — became, in queer theory, absence (trauma caused not by external agents but by one's own psychic lack or fragmentation).[4] Second, partially unremembered calls for social transformation in the past become projected as a future either vilified for its naïve aspirations or idealized for its transformative potential. Third, the negative affects rightly attached to the social causes of trauma become reattached to queerness itself, which now is seen to produce "bad feelings" from its own death drives or impossible hopes for same-sex connection. Most such accounts focus on an abstract psychic cause or locate its origins in deep histories (nineteenth-century literature, for example) that bear little or no relation to whatever traumas might produce the current generation of critics' own bad feelings. And finally, queer theory becomes preoccupied with temporal disorder — with spectral haunting, time lags, backward feelings — in ways that bring (nearly) to the surface the trauma of forgetting and the sense of temporal disruption (of flashback, broken chronology, temporal simultaneity) that similarly characterize trauma.

In drawing these connections between post-traumatic symptoms and second-wave queer theoretical preoccupations, we do not mean to claim any particular theorist as a sufferer of personal trauma. Rather, the ubiquity of these concerns suggests a collective, generational trauma, which is not the advent of AIDS itself (which was arguably more traumatic for the first wave of critics) but the unremembering of that first traumatic shock of AIDS and the subsequent desire to purchase health through strategic unremembering. Traumatized theories, to put it simply, produce post-traumatized theories. In proposing this, we do not dismiss queer theory or its insights *because* they are traumatized (although we do reject some of its symptomatic methodologies). On the contrary, we urge a return of/ to memory as a means to resolve queer theory's persistent melancholy, to reanimate its connections with the social and rhetorical innovations of previous generations of gay and lesbian thinkers (or with a current generation that still identifies with that past), and to integrate those generations' materialist critiques into the abstracted domain of academic theory. A more direct reckoning with the past and with our desires for pastness might, we hope, produce more nuanced and self-critical forms of engagement with the present and our traumatized desires for transformed social and sexual opportunities, for queer world-making. Queers are not lacking; queers are productively abundant. Queers do not experience only shame, guilt, or grief; we also experience exuberance, defiance, pride, pleasure, giddiness, enthusiastic innocence, outrageous optimism, loyalty, and love. We are, in short, as wonderfully and complexly queer as were those in our social and rhetorical pasts.

The Crisis That Is Not (Yet) One

As discourses around AIDS shifted from issues of institutional neglect, corporate profiteering, and public phobia to bad feelings that were both universalized and internalized (majoritized and minoritized, to use Eve

Sedgwick's useful terms), queer theory, it might be said, turned the fires of activism into self-immolation (*Epistemology of the Closet,* 82–86). This image invokes a touchstone narrative of trauma theory. In the story of the burning child, the father of a dead child falls asleep while a hired man sits with the corpse. As he sleeps, the father dreams that the child comes to him and calls for help as he is burning. The father awakens to discover that the hired man has in fact dropped off to sleep, allowing a lit candle to fall onto and burn the body. For Cathy Caruth, the story is a lesson in the belatedness of trauma: one realizes that one has survived trauma only after the fact, and therefore one's experience of trauma is always a fragmented and ambivalent memory. Caruth's insights into how trauma mingles memory and presence has important consequences for queer theory and AIDS narrative. If memory and presence overlap in the context of trauma, then to disavow memory, to "forget" the crisis of AIDS, is to necessarily alienate oneself from the possibility of presence as well. Queer theory's repeated articulations of "absence" — of the lack of a self-present and coherent subject with psychic unity capable of happiness — might be read as traces of such disavowed memories — memories of a historical loss and of a lost history. In the context of Caruth's analysis, absence- or rupture-based queer theory is the sleeping father, refusing to awaken not to the original trauma of the child's death, which, like deaths from AIDS, cannot be recuperated after the fact, but to the second-order trauma of not having listened *in time* to the ethical demands of memory.

Lest we turn "trauma theory" into yet another universalizing abstraction, however, we should note that AIDS is a trauma with a difference. For Caruth, belatedness is intrinsic to trauma: because the mind has no previous story through which to make sense of an unprecedented horror, the event is internalized *as* absence, generating the fragmentation and temporal disjointedness that often characterize post-traumatic testimony.[5] With AIDS, however, the trauma comes not from a lack of stories to convert loss into narrative (the long historical span of the epidemic ensures a horrifying number of such accounts) but from an abundance of memory confronting a technology of forgetting that forces unremembering upon those striving, in the face of many deaths, to retain a broader narrative of a continuity of cultural transmission.

The unremembering of AIDS may be related to its construction as a "crisis," a term (from the Greek verb "to decide") that asserts a swift move toward resolution imposed by a choice in ideals, beliefs, or strategies. While there are good reasons for constructing AIDS this way (some of which we discuss later), this model too often imposes as the *only* choice a chronologically ordered, unambivalent, and conciliatory memory narrative in which something bad is quickly repaired or ruthlessly replaced. In a psychological model, the patient "in crisis" acts — with the help of experts — to replace "unhealthy" (enraged, desiring, disjointed, perverse) patterns of actions or emotions with new ones. From this perspective, to choose the old over the new, the disordered over the chronologically progressive, ambivalence and desire over victimization and reconciliation, interpersonal struggle over individualizing psychic "ownership," is to be "locked" in the past, doomed to "acting out" (kin to AIDS activists "acting up") rather than the normative progression implied by "working through."[6] The imperative to "work through" crisis often prescribes amnesia as a prophylactic against contagious and diseased memory, as when Gabriel Rotello (as discussed in chapter 1) insisted that the necessary cure for those "so traumatized by their past as gay men" that they could not agree to sexual abstinence should be "a complete break with the past" ("Sex Clubs and Bathhouses"). For Rotello, trauma, far from bringing its own forgetting, is caused by excessive memory, the "cure" for which is a prophylactic unremembering that will bring gay men into a reparative "normalcy." The highly unstable divisions commentators like Rotello assert between sex and normalcy, traumatic memory and therapeutic forgetting, generate a crisis of social location for gay men that became a second-stage trauma.

Of course, some gay men resisted prophylactic unremembering, refusing the sexual normalization that took the AIDS crisis as its cover. As Douglas Crimp notes, "What many of us have lost is a culture of sexual possibilities: back rooms, tea rooms, bookstores, movie houses, and baths; the trucks, the pier, the ramble, the dunes. Sex was everywhere for us, and everything we wanted to venture" (*Melancholia and Moralism*, 140). Crimp clearly hasn't forgotten, nor has he saturated his memories with the shaming accusation that Rotello puts on memories of the sexual revolution. "Because this violence also desecrates the memories of our dead," Crimp argues, "we rise in anger to vindicate them. For many of us, mourning *becomes* militancy" (137). Crimp powerfully articulates a coherent account of traumatic loss, which he places at the core of militant activism. Whereas for Rotello memory brings paralysis and unremembering healthful progress, for Crimp memory brings radical action for a nonnormative present, while unremembering brings normative paralysis.

Radical deployments of memory such as Crimp's faced two obstacles, however, the first of which, arising from the internalizing, individualizing, and universalizing conceptions of (post-)Freudian melancholy, becomes evident in Crimp's manifesto, "Mourning and Militancy." Crimp begins by placing blame for traumatic loss on "ruthless interference with our bereavement," which imposed on gay memory "the violence of silence and omission almost as impossible to endure as the violence of unleashed hatred and outright murder" (*Melancholia and Moralism*, 137). Not long after naming the external agents of a second-stage trauma, Crimp concedes that "militancy might arise from conscious conflicts *within* mourning itself" (139). That subtle shift introduces an ambivalence that gets more pronounced as the essay progresses: Is the conflict *within* mourning (contained within the process of grief, and hence an effect of gay men's psychic ambivalence) or between mourning and those who would "interfere" with its processes? Initially, Crimp allows both to exist simultaneously, claiming, "When, in mourning our ideal, we meet with the same opprobrium as when mourning our dead, we incur a different order of psychic distress, since the memories of our pleasures are already fraught with ambivalence" (140). Freud notes, however, the ambivalence of melancholy leads to self-abuse on the part of the melancholic, who blames himself for situations he formerly recognized as existing outside himself. The ambivalence of melancholy, for Freud, results from an internalization, which renders "the ego itself . . . poor and empty" because the external world was impoverished — empty of the kinds of opportunity represented by the lost sex culture Crimp begins by naming — not because of ambivalence intrinsic to melancholic desire itself. Crimp becomes a Freudian melancholic, translating external forces that would "interfere" with gay memory into a loss-producing ambivalence within gay mourning itself.

The danger comes when Crimp turns the resulting "poor and empty" ego into a universal queer psyche. Social conflict over the status of gay memory thus gives way to "a fundamental fact of psychic life: violence is also self-inflicted" (146). "Unconscious conflict can mean that we may make decisions—or fail to make them—whose results may be deadly too," Crimp contends, adding, "And the rage we direct against [New York City health commissioner] Stephen Joseph, justified as it is, may function as the very mechanism of our disavowal, whereby we convince ourselves that we are making all the decisions we need to make," blinding us to "our terror, our guilt, and our profound sadness" (149). Without denying the insight of Crimp's analysis (self-inflicted ambivalence may well account for the "wrong decisions" that lead, for instance, to the rising rate of HIV infection among young gay men), his account of ambivalence threatens to erase, through psychic universalism and internalized conflict, the possibility of social contestation (militancy) over the status and public enactment of queer memory (mourning). Turning activist rage into terror, guilt, and sadness (as well as vice versa), Crimp shows how the erasure of social enactments of memory in the AIDS crisis generates the archive of negative affect that some queer theory takes up, posttraumatically, as the universal queer state.

While the internalizations of conflict into psychic ambivalence run one risk, the opposite gesture—turning history into a progressive narrative with no ambivalence at all—proves equally risky. In a 1988 speech, Vito Russo assured fellow demonstrators, "Someday, the AIDS crisis will be over. Remember that. And when that day comes, when that day has come and gone, there'll be people alive on this earth—gay people and straight people, men and women, black and white—who will hear the story that once there was a terrible disease in this country and all over the world, and that a brave group of people stood up and fought and, in some cases, gave their lives, so that other people might live and be free" ("Why We Fight"). Russo's rhetoric draws its power from a utopian prolepsis, allowing those struggling for survival against terrible odds to rest, if only momentarily, in the fictiveness of a time when a grief-stricken past will dissipate into a hagiographic and liberated future. It also promises, as David Román notes, that in the future AIDS will be "actually already a historical memory for those living after the fact" ("Remembering AIDS," 282). Román rightly admires Russo's "ability to place his own memories within a collective experience" (282), thereby building and inspiring a political entity. Russo's impetus toward collectivity is well worth remarking in the face of the de-generational unremembering that has prevented Russo's promise of AIDS's vital memory from coming true. The question for us, however, is why Russo's enabling prediction has failed to come true.

Part of the trouble comes from Russo's reliance on conventional conceptions of what it means to "remember." In his speech, "Why We Fight," memory seems to be a transparent relay between a factually self-evident past and a value-stable future, in which those remembering play no ethical or creative role. The problem with this account, as Russo acknowledges, is that *interest*—the fact that some go on "as though we weren't living through some sort of nightmare" while others "hear the screams of the people who are dying and their cries for help"—suggests that the present is not a neutral space of transmission but rather comprises competing claims to justice, in which memory, created or disavowed from those positions of interest, plays a crucial role.

Read carefully, however, the promise of remembering held out in Russo's speech is lodged in his opening line. The first sentence of Russo's speech does not promise an end to AIDS but an end to "crisis"—a locution that implies a beginning to remembering. When activists named AIDS a crisis, they indicated its profoundly *traumatic* nature, meaning not only the horrors of the syndrome itself but also its existence outside and against the apparently seamless temporality of Russo's inspiring promise. For despite the model of decisive conclusion implied by "crisis" in the psychic life of both individuals and collectives, in fact the time and place of crisis are revisited again and again with the focus not on the satisfaction of resolution but on the trauma associated with the original event (think of the role the "Cuban missile crisis" played in subsequent American politics). To embrace the countertemporal traumatic effects of crisis is to break from the predictable sequencing of both memory and narrative (memory *as* narrative). Trauma survivors are often characterized as temporal stutterers, starting again and again, struggling to give chronological order to stubbornly disjointed affects and events. By insisting on the AIDS crisis as trauma—and by encouraging the work of memory in that trauma—we confront the imperatives toward unremembering that misrecognize "moving beyond" memory as a sign of health. Unremembering is not a sign that a crisis is over; it is the beginning of a trauma all its own. We insist on the right to memory without necessitating the imposition of normative values, redemptive chronology, or prophylactic forgetting.

The language of crisis, moreover, insists on the *social* location of AIDS, providing an external object on which to direct our anger and our sadness rather than internalizing our mourning into negative affects we supposedly carry, like scars of past burnings, at the core of our irremediably sad and shameful selves. Accepting the traumatic implications of living through crisis allows us to understand queer memory as neither transparent nor recuperative but rather, as Caruth suggests, as a register of belatedness. Understanding that we are awakening too late to the loss of those who died from AIDS and the cultures they created is not an occasion for self-blame. No one could have had narratives in place with which to anticipate the horrors of AIDS and its effects. The work of remembering is to provide those narratives, stories that might offer creative ways to renew our sense of mutual responsibility and reinvigorate forms of post-essentialist (including the "essence" of negative affect) inventive pleasure.

To call for more memory of/in crisis in the name of creativity and pleasure may seem counterintuitive, but memory can occasion joy and progressive invention as much as grief. Here we can return to Caruth's analysis of the tale of the dead child who calls out that he is burning. "The passing on of the child's words transmits not simply a reality that can be grasped in these words' repetition," Caruth contends, "but the ethical imperative of an awakening that has yet to occur" (*Unclaimed Experience,* 112). To awaken to one's responsibility to the past is not, then, an imperative to re-create the past exactly and transparently *as it was* but rather an invitation to ethical imagination. Awakening to a present in which one perceives "the very gap between the other's death and his own life," we inherit the opportunity for "crossing from the burning within to the burning without" (106). Following Caruth's lead, we can see that unless we respond to the cry of the past—to pastness in its extrasubjective specificity of loss—we will continue to misconstrue a burning without as a burning within, social inflictions of shame as internally abjecting drives. These misrecognitions cause us to miss our present creative capability to respond to bad feeling by generating not utopian futures or amnesic presents but *memories*. Suspended between a responsibility to the spectacular *realness* of the past and the collaborative *inventiveness* of the present, these memories will allow for creative collaboration as an activist practice against the current culture of amnesia.

Queer Theory Is Burning

Although the abstractions ("absence," "self-shattering," "the death drive," "antisociality") represented by much first-wave queer theory's turn to what Michael Snediker calls "queer pessimism" threaten to obscure the social losses at their core, those losses remain visible in the disillusionment and shame associated by de-generational unremembering with the sexual revolution (now abstracted simply as "sex"). The social losses associated throughout the late 1980s and early 1990s with "sex" were translated into rhetorical shattering, death drives, and melancholic absences detached from their historical ties and reattached to universalized psychological or ontological inevitabilities. This translation both registers and perpetuates the negative affects attached by de-generational unremembering, through AIDS, to sex and sexual culture, creating from the trauma of loss a post-trauma of forgetting. Leo Bersani's 1987 essay "Is the Rectum a Grave?" with its essentializing and universalizing claims about sexuality deployed against "the rhetoric of sexual liberation in the '60s and '70s" (219) (as analyzed in chapter 1) is an important example of such translations, in part because it bears traces of the social origins of its abstracted (and very influential) claims about sex's anticommunalism. Written to help explain the appallingly cruel and paranoid treatment of AIDS sufferers early in the epidemic, the essay risked, in Bersani's words, "the pain of embracing, at least provisionally, a homophobic representation of homosexuality" (209). That context of homophobia and its provisional embrace went unacknowledged and unremembered in the reiteration and extrapolation of Bersani's claims (that camp is unsexy, that sexual camaraderie is a myth, that penetration is shattering, that "most people don't like sex"), which, though dubious, were rarely challenged from within the ranks of first-wave queer theorists and in many cases were rehearsed as the truth of queerness.

The effects of Bersani's claims — both in terms of their content and the unremembering of their context as a project to understand homophobia — become clear in the summer 2007 issue of *South Atlantic Quarterly*, "After

Sex?" (Halley and Parker). The issue's title succinctly captures the conversion of loss (to be "after" in the sense of "post-" is to have moved beyond the moment when sex was possible, much less likable) into absence (to be "after sex" in the sense of looking for sex is to assume that one is in a state of desire for what one does not have); in the first account, the disappearance of sex is chronological, in the second, ontological. This shift from historical loss to ontological absence has generated a preoccupation with negative affect—of bad feelings come loose from their historical occasions—that can be seen in the titles of the essays in the "After Sex?" issue: "Starved," "Lonely," "Glad to Be Unhappy," "Queer Theory: Postmortem," "Disturbing Sexuality," "Post Sex: On Being Too Slow, Too Stupid, Too Soon." Even when ironic, these titles reflect Heather Love's assertion that the archive of queer feelings is a tour de force of depressive symptoms: "nostalgia, regret, shame, despair, *ressentiment,* passivity, escapism, self-hatred, withdrawal, bitterness, defeatism, and loneliness" (*Feeling Backward,* 4). It is debatable whether this catalog of bad feelings has been, as Love claims, the primary "corporeal and psychic" (4) response to antigay violence, including the assault on queer memory described earlier. The pride, exuberance, shamelessness, defiance, purposefulness, enthusiasm, hilarity, and joy of the Gay Pride movement and the sexual revolution (discussed in the following section) would constitute an alternative "archive." Focusing on negative feelings is not a psychic or historical inevitability, but a *choice,* and while that focus provides a useful counterbalance to the uncritical "pride" and liberationist romanticism of some earlier rhetoric, much second-wave queer theory since the mid-1990s has privileged pessimistic affects in ways that not only seem, in Snediker's words, "strangely routinized" (*Queer Optimism,* 4) but that erase the sexual culture of the 1970s while normalizing the traumatized loss of the post-AIDS generation. We understand these bad feelings as a poignant surfacing of grief without an object, that object having been made unnamable first by the conservative assault on memory, then by mainstream media's erasure of AIDS from its daily rehearsal of national crises, and finally by first-wave queer theory's own translation of historical loss into ontological absence or fragmentation.

One particularly sophisticated example of how second-wave queer theory enacts a post-traumatic narrative that effaces historical conflict in favor of psychic abstraction and negative affects can be found in a forum on the "antisocial thesis in queer theory" in the May 2006 issue of *PMLA*. Here four scholars were asked to examine the "antisocial thesis" derived from Bersani, which asserts that queer sex epitomizes the self-shattering, anticommunitarian death drive that queers have historically represented within Western culture. As part of that forum, Lee Edelman and Judith Halberstam push the antisocial thesis further, expanding its political (or, conversely, antipolitical, the two terms seeming, vertiginously, to describe similar affects) efficacy (or, again, antiefficacy).

For Halberstam, queer theory's archive—totalized as "the gay male archive"—proves disappointingly narrow. Focused on Marcel Proust, Virginia Woolf, Bette Midler, Andy Warhol, Broadway musicals, and Judy Garland (among others), gay men, according to Halberstam, have failed to notice the realpolitiks in a more radically antiracist and counternormative archive comprising Valerie Solanas (Warhol's would-be assassin, whose Society for Cutting Up Men [SCUM] manifesto was sponsored into print by Vivian Gornick as an expression of a frankly homophobic form of feminism),[7] a number of cartoon characters (Wallace and Gromit, the fish in *Finding Nemo*, SpongeBob, and Hothead Paisan), artists who work in cartoony styles (the apolitical Nicole Eisenman, and Deborah Cass, whose invocation of cartoons is intended as a homage to Warhol), and—oddly, given Halberstam's contempt for the "gay male archive's" focus on "favored canonical writers"—Toni Morrison ("The Politics of Negativity," 824).[8] Leaving aside the stereotypical characterization of gay men as exclusively devoted to the dandyish affects of "fatigue, ennui, boredom, ironic distancing, indirectness, arch dismissal, insincerity, and camp," what is noteworthy here is Halberstam's insistence, through her countercanon, that we broaden queer theory's affective range to include "rage, rudeness, anger, spite, impatience, intensity, mania, sincerity, earnestness, overinvestment, incivility, and brutal honesty" (824).

We endorse calls to infuse queer theory with more rage and sincerity. What's intriguing here, though, is the seeming incongruity of the affects Halberstam describes. The aggressiveness of rage, rudeness, anger, spite, impatience, intensity, mania, and incivility seems to have little in common with the quieter and gentler affects of sincerity, earnestness, and an honesty that need not be brutal. These affective sets are less incongruous, though, when considered in the context of trauma, where both coexist in the survivor who manifests earnest and sincere honesty (a determination to get stories "right," to provide accurate chronology, to appear more transparently sincere than artful, lest one be accused of producing "false memories"), as well as the spiteful rudeness of "acting out" in the absence of narrative credibility or accessible memory. Frustrated by their inability to provide the transparent sincerity they wish to convey or to name the object of their anger, trauma survivors act out through inarticulate rage, obsessive repetition, and violent incivility. Understood in terms of trauma's simultaneous production of sincerity and rage, overinvestment and incivility, Halberstam's list of seemingly incongruous affects makes more sense. And if we understand that trauma survivors are often characterized as children, who also combine earnest honesty and frustrated rage and who are also seen as existing in an early stage of the trajectory toward maturity, we can understand why Halberstam centers her preferred archive on cartoons and children's movies.

Halberstam's contribution to the PMLA forum is emblematic of second-wave post-traumatic narrative in the way it casts the traumatized past as an idealized future. "If we want to make the antisocial turn in queer theory," Halberstam concludes, "we must be willing to turn away from the comfort zone of polite exchange to embrace a truly political negativity, one that promises, this time, to fail, to make a mess, to fuck shit up, to be loud, unruly, impolite, to breed resentment, to bash back, etc." (824). Striking in this passage is Halberstam's location of her idealized affects in the future (her urging that "we must" do certain things implies that they're *not* being done now, that "the promise" of "a truly political negativity" exists only futurally, *as* a promise that displaces the present). Her phrase "this time" thus signifies not here and now but a future when her idealized affects will be taken up, a present yet to come that will not need, as the present and the past apparently do, a supplemental future. Halberstam's piece participates actively in the unremembering of the past. To acknowledge the rage, incivility, sincere overinvestment, and willingness to fuck shit up of those who created gloryholes in public restrooms, who unfurled banners from the balcony of the New York Stock Exchange, who resisted arrest, issued proclamations calling for universal health care and an end to imperialist wars, blocked traffic, threw bricks, changed voting districts, threw pies at notorious bigots on live TV—to acknowledge *this* past would not only complicate homophobic constructions of "the gay male archive" and its bored and stylized ennui, it would show that the future for which Halberstam is waiting has always been right behind her. The past occluded by Halberstam—a past that combines sincerity and rage, honesty and incivility—often appears in survivor narratives in the figure of the child. Trauma survivors often express deep ambivalences toward children and childhood, especially when childhood is the scene of trauma and when the child represents a hopeful innocence that will be redeemed from a traumatic past in some unspecified future (once one has "worked through" trauma and reclaimed the "child within"). The futural child can thus become, in traumatic narratives, a figure of both desire and rage, of rage *because* of an unacknowledged desire. In his contribution to the PMLA Forum, Lee Edelman offers a sarcastic parody of queer humanism represented by the figure of the child. Rather than refuting Halberstam's charge that gay men are not socially engaged, Edelman expresses a wish for *more* disengagement, lampooning those who,

> happy to earn their applause . . . by putting the puppet of humanism through its passion play once again . . . lead in a hymn to the Futurch even while dressed in heretical drag. Delightfully drugged by the harmony, the freedom from harm, that their harmonies promise, they induce us all to nod along, persuaded that we, like their puppet, on which most humanities teaching depends, shall also eventually overcome, for knowledge, understanding, and progress must, in the fullness of time, set us free. ("Antagonism," 821)

What Edelman here mocks as "the Futurch" is embodied in the child and its deceptive capacity to symbolize a transformative future. It's significant that, in this passage, deluded humanists shift from being puppeteers (adults who put the puppet "of humanism through its passion play") to being children (the audience for puppet shows, nodding along in unanalyzed pleasure). What begins as a condemnation of the alluring adult ends by condemning the seduced child. Children, in this scene, perpetually reenact their seduction (the "passion play" is performed "once again"), combining in the reiterative present a past that cannot be abandoned and a future that, hopelessly seeking freedom from its "passion play," can never be achieved. Hating that child for having put his faith in a violently disillusioning future (while never quite abandoning that child's faith, now represented in an equally idealized future with no more alluring passion plays), Edelman enacts an ambivalence toward the past and the future (the past *as* the future, innocent trust in the pleasure principle now recast as an equally innocent faith in the death drive). The only "good" kid, the only knowing queer, would therefore be the one who could know *ahead of time* the repeated presence of death, a child with no future, a traumatized child, which is to say, Edelman-as-theorist.

Given that Edelman stages his own passion play of reiterated trauma against an over-optimistic queer humanism, we might understand his figural child as representing a collective past, a previous innocence seduced by optimism only to find that its future of promised liberation has been foreclosed by insistently shattering death (drives). The hated but desired child (hated *because* desired, giving ambivalence to Edelman's injunction to "fuck children") can be said to be liberationist discourse itself, which in this construction promised a time that will "set us free" only to produce the shattering disillusionment of AIDS. It is worth recalling that the sexual culture of the 1970s and the gay men who participated in it were characterized in de-generational diatribes as *infantile:* narcissistic, pleasure driven, and irresponsible, in a state of perpetually arrested development. The liberal "child" of futural democracy as the object of Edelman's critique is the temporal twin of the neoconservative vision of the gay past as locked in a permanent state of the infantile uncanny. Bifurcated, like gay culture generally, between a disavowed past and an unworthy future, neither child is allowed to grow, like Kathryn Bond Stockton's queer child, sideways into the present.

In their elisions of past and future, their understanding of both in relation to the affects of childhood, their love and disgust for the fucked (over) child, Halberstam and Edelman produce second-wave queer theory as a post-traumatic survival narrative. Much of the trauma in both essays is a never-quite-achieved unremembering, which, we have argued, haunts second-wave queer theory. Even efforts to supplant "a faltering antirelational model of queer theory with a queer utopianism" that highlights "a renewed interest in social theory" built "on a well-established tradition of critical idealism," as José Esteban Muñoz puts it in his contribution to the PMLA Forum, accepts an impoverished vision of the legacy from the gay past, positing the antisocial as "the gay white man's last stand" ("Thinking beyond Antirelationality," 825). Queerness in this view is located only in the future: "for queerness to have any value whatsoever, it must be considered visible only on the horizon" (825). We offer the alternative of memory as another powerful way to resist "a totalizing and naturalizing idea of the present" (825) from *within* the present. Memory, moreover, does not require us to site utopian difference on an ever-receding horizon, a strategy that risks deferring utopia in just the way Muñoz rightly criticizes negativity for doing. Whether a utopian ideal is foreclosed by the death drive or put beyond reach by an ever-receding futural horizon seems, on an important level, of less importance than the shared result: the presumed unachievability in the present of the ideal. Queer theory has frequently promised more — has promised, in fact, the capacity to make new worlds. That promise is deeply rooted in our cultural past, and if we want queer theory to make good on its promises, we best not forget it.

"We Articulate Cocksucker Values": Remembering the Sexual Revolution

The campaign of unremembering that followed the onset of AIDS targeted the so-called sexual revolution of the late 1960s and 1970s. This episode was not completely forgotten but retrospectively transformed from a period of creative sexual and social experimentation and self-expression into a reckless sexual free-for-all of heartless promiscuity that caused the widespread dissemination of HIV/AIDS and hindered efforts to bring gay men to practices that would stem the tide of infection. To resist this dynamic, we might remember the sexual revolution as an *intellectual* movement, a collective theoretical articulation of critical practice centered on the embodied nexus of rageful challenge, hopeful invention, and erotic liberation. This self-understanding constituted the meaning(s) of the sexual freedoms of the period, although it now risks disappearing from both histories and theories of sexuality.

The intellectual freedoms generated during the 1960s and 1970s, which were essential to subsequent gay, lesbian, and queer theory, were unremembered through both right-wing narratives of sexual excess reaping its just reward and through the (mostly academic) left's assaults on the communitarian ethos of so-called identity politics and subsequent appeals to the future to provide the values and affects unremembered in the past. By calling for a distinctively queer praxis yet to come or by placing

that praxis within the psychic drives that efface historically situated pastness, much queer theory, as we discussed earlier, repressed the prior existence of that theoretical praxis as *having already been.* The "rage, rudeness,
anger, spite, impatience, intensity, mania, sincerity, earnestness, overinvestment, incivility, and brutal honesty" Halberstam calls for, and the
disavowal of a reproductive futurity Edelman calls for, for instance, have
already existed in the past. By framing such calls as innovation, queer
theory grounded itself in a misrecognition of what was, in fact, *renovation,* a reshaping of pastness to meet the needs of the present. This unremembering, in turn, contributed to a sense of absence or melancholy
that theorists misconstrued as a timeless feature of the queer condition
rather than recognizing as traumatically historical.

The cost here is not simply the wasted effort of wheel reinvention but
the loss of some of the most affectively and imaginatively rich and daring contributions to the queer intellectual tradition. As Simon Watney
observes in *Imagine Hope,* the "generous libertarian traditions of Gay Liberation have gradually ossified into a frozen leftist orthodoxy of ghastly,
dour moralism and furious self-righteousness" (268), with academics,
especially in the United States, limited to an "arid domain of compulsory
theoretical abstraction, with its rigid orthodoxies and its remorseless anti-
idealism" (250). Noting that in twelve anthologies of gay and lesbian academic essays published in the 1990s, only 25 of 233 articles took up some
aspect of HIV/AIDS, while in three special "queer" issues of respected
academic journals, three of thirty-nine articles were about HIV/AIDS
(245), Watney blames this oversight on the anti-identity (and hence anticommunitarian) ethos of queer theory in the academy, "in which studies
are herded through a curriculum that in effect often denies the validity
or authenticity of any kind of communitarian or collective lesbian or gay
culture or politics" (251), although those collective cultures, in the context of AIDS, "provide the most reliable forms of resistance and mutual
protection" (250). Thus, Watney contends, queer theory reproduced the
competitive individualism of the Thatcher–Reagan period "it ostensi-
bly opposed" (17). Our contention is that the dour ossification Watney
describes is haunted by (barely) repressed memories of a more vibrant
and daring intellectual moment. Our hope is that this unremembering is
beginning to be reversed, leading to renewed intellectual and rhetorical

vivacity within queer theory. To contribute to that change, we turn now to what the writers of the sexual revolution might still teach us.

Although the "sexual revolution" flourished in the United States mostly between the late 1960s and the late 1970s, its intellectual roots can be traced to the publication of the Kinsey Reports on male and female sexuality (1948 and 1951, respectively) and continuing through the publication in 1951 of Wilhelm Reich's *The Sexual Revolution*, in 1955 of Herbert Marcuse's *Eros and Civilization*, and in 1966 of Norman O. Brown's *Love's Body*. From these works, intellectuals of the late 1960s and 1970s — among whom we might name Jill Johnston, Audre Lorde, Carl Wittman, Gayle Rubin, Dennis Altman, Erica Jong, Boyd McDonald, Lawrence Lipton, Amber Hollibaugh, Paul Goodman, Cherríe Moraga, Harry Hay, Pat Califia, Charley Shively, Kate Millett, and John Rechy — drew a distinctive picture of the radically innovative and counternormative nature of sex, sexuality, and eroticism in everyday life. Out of the oppression they experienced came not just bad feelings but also keen insight and a vibrant determination to resist and to change the sexual, social, and intellectual mores of midcentury America. "The sexual outlaws — boy-lovers, sadomasochists, prostitutes, and transpeople, among others — have an especially rich knowledge of the prevailing system of sexual hierarchy and of how sexual controls are exercised," Gayle Rubin proclaimed in 1981, concluding that this knowledge endowed these queer constituencies with "a great deal to contribute to the reviving radical debate on sexuality" ("The Leather Menace," 297). In 1978, Audre Lorde went so far as to place erotic sensation at the origin of the will to dissent, claiming, "The erotic is a measure between the beginnings of our sense of self and the chaos of our strongest feelings. It is an internal sense of satisfaction to which, once we have experienced it, we know we can aspire" ("Uses of the Erotic," 167). Writers like Rubin and Lorde understood their work not only in terms of criticism, challenge, or confrontation but also as an expansion of imaginative potential in which sex and eroticism opened new forms of embodiment, relationality, representation, and world-making. It is these qualities of "exhilaration, the sense of freedom and the utopian impulse that underlay it," as Jeffrey Escoffier notes in the introduction to his useful (though underused) anthology of writings from the sexual revolution, that are "often forgotten today" (*Sexual Revolution,* xii). In characterizing the problem as one of forgetting, Escoffier places memory—and the lack thereof—at the heart of an affective and imaginative poverty in contemporary thinking about sexuality.

The sexual revolution was, first and foremost, an assault on social and sexual conventions, from monogamy, marriage, hypocritical propriety, and possessive reproduction to more generalized systems of coercive normalcy, surplus labor, abusive power, and social divisions brought about by policed definitions of identity. Far from efforts to reify a monolithic sexual identity or to segregate sexuality from broader social operations of power and resistance, the agendas of sexual liberation were often insistently coalitional, as in the "Statement of Purpose" Harry Hay penned in 1969 for the Gay Liberation Front of Los Angeles, in which he declared, "We are in total opposition to America's white racism, to poverty, hunger, the systematic destruction of our patrimony; we oppose the rich getting richer, the poor getting poorer, and are in total opposition to wars of aggression and imperialism, whoever pursues them. We support the demands of Blacks, Chicanos, Orientals, Women, Youth, Senior Citizens, and others demanding their full rights as human beings. We join in their struggle, and shall actively seek coalition to pursue these goals" (*Radically Gay,* 176–77). Two years later, a joint statement from the organizations Third World Gay Revolution (Chicago) and Gay Liberation Front (Chicago) called for those who saw the "potential for love with equality and freedom" to become "a force for everyone's ultimate liberation,"

a tool to break down enforced heterosexuality, sex roles, the impoverished categories of straight, gay, and bisexual, male supremacy, programming of children, ownership of children, the nuclear family, monogamy, possessiveness, exclusiveness of "love," insecurity, jealousy, competition, privilege, individual isolation, ego-tripping, power-tripping, money-tripping, people as property, people as machines, rejection of the body, repression of emotion, anti-eroticism, authoritarian, anti-human religion, conformity, regimentation, polarization of "masculine" and "feminine," categorizations of male and female emotions, abilities, interests, clothing, etc., fragmentation of the self by these outlines, isolation and elitism of the arts, uniform standards of beauty, dependency on leaders, unquestioning submission to authority, power hierarchies, caste, racism, militarism, imperialism, national chauvinism, cultural chauvinism, domination, exploitation, division, inequality, and repression as the cultural and politico-economic norms, all manifestations of non-respect and non-love for what is human (not to mention animals and plants) — maybe even up to private property and the state. ("Gay Revolution and Sex Roles," 258)

The issues addressed in this statement — the insufficiency of identity categories, the inadequacy of monogamous marriage and the reproductive family, the need to resist conceptions of love as competitive possessiveness, the devastating and far-reaching consequences of power hierarchies, and the broad suppression of love and respect — are taken up again and again in the writings of the period, pointing to a widely held collective materialist focus on the expansive affects and inventive self-understandings of sexual subjectivity that exceed and disrupt the regimes of competitive capitalism, essentialized identity, and normalized hierarchy that structured the lives of Americans at midcentury.

Such challenges focused on what Lawrence Lipton in 1965 called "the old sexways, the traditional morality of monogamous marriage," that had grown to "an advanced state of decay" (From *The Erotic Revolution,* 185). As Harry Hay put the problem in 1970, "Our vain-hallowed culture is slowly sinking into a veritable kitchen midden of obscenely generated *unexamined assumptions,* learned by rote, inherited without question, and having not one shred of a basis for possible justification in the modern world" (*Radically Gay,* 193). "In this hell of Anomie," Hay observed, "we of the Homosexual Minority have been reduced to semi-conscious rudderless wanderers, driven like sheep to conform to social patterns which atrophied our perceptions and shredded our souls, beset on every side by the bacilli of — to us — alien value-judgments which riddled the very sinews of our Dream" (197). To free us from our bondage to decrepit sexways and naturalized normativity, an anonymous writer for *Fag Rag* called in 1971 for the proliferation of "cocksucker values" embodied in promiscuous acts of nonreproductive sex in public. "Any essential part of any program for those who cherish freedom must be to trash the nuclear family," he claimed, adding, "so conceived, every cock sucked is an act of liberation" ("Cocksucker," 515). This writer was probably Charley Shively, a frequent contributor to *Fag Rag,* whose 1974 "Indiscriminate Promiscuity as an Act of Revolution" contended that "faggots" (precursor of the recuperative "queer") are uniquely qualified "to break away from the existing power structure and search out new alternatives. The nuclear family is the foundation stone of all that is established" (257). In order to create an alternative social foundation, Shively argued that eroticism had to be radically expanded, "sexualized, changed, revolutionized." Adding, "The alienation most of us feel most of the time is most pronounced in our most intimate institutions — the 'family' of social units in which we live" (262), Shively offered "cocksucker values" not as "a utopian fantasy, but as a way for making change, a way rooted in the actual social experience of faggots — a way tied deeply into centuries of suffering and experience" (261). Indiscriminate promiscuity, Shively promised, would bring about a radical erosion of the borders between public and private, corporeality and collectivity, sexuality and sociality. Effacing such deeply ingrained divisions, "our sexuality makes us revolutionary" (257).

While sexuality might efface most boundaries and divisions, there was one sex radicals sought to maintain and strengthen: that between erotics and economics. For Shively and others of this period, radical insight derived from their alienation from conventions that shaped love, eroticism, and social attachment in the image of competitive capitalism. Noting that Americans treat intimacy the way they treat private property, Shively stated, "Everyone is constantly hoarding people and love" (263). Rather than making sex "an in-between activity," Shively encouraged his readers to "make every action sexual," thereby undermining "capitalist decadence," which separates business and pleasure. In such a world, Shively concluded, "our sexuality would not 'drag' us down or wear us out for the tasks of building a totally free society. Our sexuality would be that society" (262). Pushing for what he called sexual socialism, Shively imagined anonymous promiscuity overthrowing an evaluative economics oriented toward the values of normative masculinity, too often translated by gay men into discriminatory hierarchies of penis or muscle size, age, machismo, and so on. Capitalism had especially injurious consequences, Shively argued, for working-class and ethnic men who are forced to perform conventional masculinity and hence to disavow not only homosexuality but intimacy in general (258). "Everything boils down to *inequality*," according to Shively; "We live in a culture/economy where all things are measured and sold; any inequality is counted and counts against you" (260–61). Shively's response to commodification is socialist not only because it rests on an analysis of unequally distributed capital but also because it calls for collective response rather than for governmental reform. Faggots who wait for state-granted equality or even legal recognition, according to Shively, are dangerously naïve about the extent that state power relies on masculinist hierarchies. "In calling for a socialist society," he asserted, "we do not ask some party or state to suddenly give something to us. . . . We don't want something, we want everything" (263).

Others in the generation of 1970s sexual radicals echoed Shively's analysis. Dennis Altman in 1971 put forth a Marxist critique of stingy intimacy, asserting that "compulsory monogamy and possessiveness" are direct outgrowths of "our cult of acquisitiveness that makes us feel that love need be rationed" ("Liberation," 638). "'In America,' Kate Millett has said, 'you can either fuck or shake hands,'" Altman reported, "and this sums up the situation. The ability to feel, to hold, to embrace, to take comfort from the warmth of other human beings is sadly lacking" (635). Endorsing "a new sense of play and spontaneity" as a counterforce to accumulations rationalized by false scarcity, Altman pictured gays and lesbians as pioneers of what Norman O. Brown called "'a science of enjoyment rather than a science of accumulation'" ("Liberation," 636), an ethos exemplified by Pat Califia, who in 1979 stated, "I am interested in something ephemeral, pleasure, not in economic control or forced reproduction" ("A Secret Side," 534).

Recognizing the economic sources of "the trouble with normal," Jill Johnston in 1973 noted how "puritan ethical appeals to the moral correctness of doing things that are worthwhile by their difficulty and hard labor through delayed gratification of real instincts, or uniting with self," have naturalized heteronormativity. Johnston asserted, "There's no conceivable equality between two species in a relation in which one of the two has been considerably weakened in all aspects of her being over so long a period of historical time." The "normal" state of reproductive heterosexuality, according to Johnston, can produce only a "civilized schizophrenia" generative of "pseudo-normalcy" ("The Myth of the Myth," 506–7). More optimistically, Amber Hollibaugh and Cherríe Moraga in 1981 called for a "heterosexuality beyond heterosexism" ("What We're Rollin' Around in Bed With," 539), in which straights joined queers in rejecting the commodification of the body as an acquirable possession or a coerced means of production. This imperative to contest conventional power dynamics by embracing the body's androgynous, polymorphous state of flawed diversity echoes Altman's call, a decade earlier, for an erotics that celebrates "the funkiness of the body" in opposition to "the plastic, odorless, hairless and blemishless creations of *Playboy* and its homosexual equivalents" ("Liberation," 638).

Alternatives to the conventional commodification of the "hairless blemishless" body were enacted in the 1970s and early 1980s in S/M subcultures as well as the subsequently much-maligned gay "clone" culture. These movements generated serious erotic pleasure in the appropriation — even parody — of styles associated with what Gayle Rubin in 1981 called the "entire right-wing program" of "military build-up, family reconstruction, anti-communism, and enforced sexual conformity" ("The Leather Menace," 268). Rubin, mocking the mainstream fears of a queer "leather menace," observed that normalcy can be naturalized only through "frequent recourse to terror," producing "a vast vague pool of nameless horror" (267). The coercive system of what John Rechy called "legally sanctioned sadism" (*The Sexual Outlaw*, 102) was appropriated and performed in S/M, which, Califia argued,

> recognizes the sexual underpinnings of our system, and seeks to reclaim them. There's an enormous hard-on beneath the priest's robe, the cop's uniform, the president's business suit, the soldier's khakis. But the phallus is powerful only as long as it is concealed, elevated to the level of a symbol, never exposed or used in literal fucking. In an S&M context, the uniforms and roles and dialogue become a parody of authority, a challenge to it, a recognition of its secret sexual nature. ("A Secret Side," 534–35)

Queer sadomasochists, according to Califia, "select all the most frightening, disgusting, or unacceptable activities and transmute them into pleasure. We make use of all the forbidden symbols and all the disowned emotions" (528). Or, as Shively more whimsically stated, "Instead of being awed and fearing priests, police, officers, sailors, marines, teachers, cardinals, jocks, soldiers, students and other 'respectables' — we want to bring them to bed with us. All the capitalist toilet training gets flushed away in many golden showers" (*Meat*, 6).

At the other end of the wide spectrum of anticonventional sexual styles and politics in the era before "queer," the Radical Faeries rejected the trappings of power manifest in S/M and clone culture, choosing instead to recall from childhood "the suddenly remembered sense of awe and wonder" in nature (Hay, *Radically Gay*, 256). The resultant "Fairy Vision" comprised, according to Harry Hay, "beautiful beckoning not-as-yet-comprehensible secret sacra" (258). For Hay and others who gathered in the Arizona desert for the first time in 1979, the Radical Faery movement promised mutual responsibility in place of the competitive depersonalization and commercialization they found in the urban gay male world. Hay's 1980 manifesto "This New Planet of Fairy-Vision" lays out a five-point process for transforming "from Hetero-imitating Gays into Radical Fairies" (255). Beginning with an effort "to reunite ourselves with the cornered, frightened, rejected little Sissy-kids we all once were" and "to recapture and restore in full honors that magick of 'being a different species perceiving a different reality,'" fairies tell "that *different* boy that he was remembered . . . loved . . . and deeply respected" and that "we now recognized that he, in true paradox, had always been the real source of our Dream, of our strength to resist, of our stubborn endurance — a strength, again in true paradox, that few Hetero Males can even begin to approach, let alone match." Following these stages, fairies can convince "that beloved little Sissy that we had experienced a full paradigm shift and that he could now come home at last to be himself in full appreciation" (255). Hay's invocation of the queer child is worth recalling for its critique of the foreclosure of intimate collectivity by normative masculinity and its proposal of a viable social alternative other than that promised by S/M. Above all, Hay's program for fairy transformation placed memory at the heart of queer collectivity. While the remembered past might be individual in name (each fairy's sissy within), the sense of "awe and wonder" recaptured through those memories and shared in the present transform traumatic memory of alienation into an enabling program of collective queer world-making.

Most important to understanding the radical potential of the sexual revolution, however, is what S/M activists and Radical Faeries shared: a critical investment in the radical redistribution of the body's pleasures both by expanding its erogenous zones beyond the genitals and by proliferating opportunities for collective pleasure. These values underpin the advocacy by many writers of the sexual revolution of cruising, anonymity, and promiscuity. Understanding the entire body and every social interaction as opportunities for pleasure, these writers posited erotics as an important antidote to the repressive logic of reserved labor and possessive monogamy, which made deferred and denied pleasure the sine qua non of loving trust and economic well-being. Making sex both accessible and available in a society starved for human contact and sensual satisfaction, promiscuity expands the body's erogenous range, taking us, one *Fag Rag* contributor argued, beyond "the sexual objectification of the cock" and toward "ear, nose, mouth, toe, tongue, knee, ass, back, arm, finger, nipple, loin, groin, and other part sucking," a corporeal democracy that would, in turn, make concepts of privacy disappear ("Cocksucker," 513, 515). Promiscuity, as Charley Shively argued, is not "some dream or fantasy." Because our bodies are "commonplace things found in every home" they can be the means of nearly ubiquitous pleasure, "the source of change and revolution" ("Indiscriminate Promiscuity," 258). Shively insisted that "the political" be revolutionary and embodied, accessible ("commonplace") and extraordinary. Promiscuity, countermanding hierarchical body values modeled on straight, white, able-bodied masculinity, would, Shively maintained, redistribute sexual pleasure to poor, ugly, disabled, uneducated, and nonwhite men who might be discriminated against in bars. "Our bodies are real," Shively insisted; "they are not some social theory, some utopian proposal; their relationship to labor, the state, the economy and consciousness is not less fundamental than the other way around" (257).

Altman similarly argued that liberation requires "a general eroticization of human life — by which I mean an acceptance of the sensuality that we all possess, and a willingness to let it imbue all personal contacts — and a move toward polymorphous perversity that includes more than reassessment of sex roles" ("Liberation," 631). More stridently, John Rechy declared in 1977, "The promiscuous homosexual is a sexual revolutionary. Every moment of his outlaw existence he confronts repressive laws, repressive 'morality'" (*The Sexual Outlaw,* 28). Rechy gives allegorical form to the opposition between public erotic pleasure and hypocritical repression when he describes being on a cruisy California beach with "some very gorgeous people" when their fun is suddenly interrupted by the appearance of a woman and a "sagging-skin man," "a small, wrinkled dinosaur . . . body hidden almost totally to the brash sun," whose eyes pointed "invisible guns." The intruding hostile figures, embodying the decay Lipton saw in the "old morality," turn out to be Ronald and Nancy Reagan (45). Faced with this ominous allegory of America's repressive future, Rechy's outlaws become fiercer, more exuberantly and defiantly promiscuous, more creative in staking out codes and spaces to enable sexual proliferation. Knowing that "each second his freedom may be ripped away arbitrarily," a promiscuous outlaw "lives fully at the brink," a psychic and physical liminality generative of "insurrectory power that can bring down their straight world" if queers "take the war openly into the streets. As long as they continue to kill us," Rechy urged, "fuck and suck on every corner! Question their hypocritical, murderous, uptight world" (31–32). "Public sex is revolution," Rechy asserts, "courageous, righteous, defiant revolution" (47).

Aggressive confrontation was one strategy; campy creativity was another. Throughout the pages of *Straight to Hell,* for instance, editor Boyd McDonald, who was reportedly inspired by Gore Vidal's character Myra Breckenridge visiting him in a dream, offered "real-life" testimony of the promiscuous, raunchy, power-saturated proliferation of pleasure occurring throughout American society. Often humorously subtitled *The U.S. Chronicle of Crimes Against Nature, The American Journal of Dick Licking, New York Review of Cocksucking* (Shively, *Meat,* 5), *Straight to Hell* applied "cocksucker values" to the foundations of normative masculinity: the church, the military, schools, sports, and commerce. Even a short list of article titles conveys something of the variety of provocations and pleasures this promised in these pages: "Youth Removes Jockey Shorts, Sits on Coach's Face," "General's Cum Cake," "Father Knows Best," "Hubby's Night Out with the Boys," "I Slept with My Nose Up His Ass," "81-Year-Old Ready and Eager," "State Trooper Nookie," "Sucks Priest in Black Jockstrap," "Takes 16 Up Ass, 14 Down Throat," "Farmer Uses Films to Seduce Hired Hands, Aged 18, 19, and 20," "The Heartbreak of Butt Pimples," "Clergyman Wipes Cop's Ass," "Three Brothers Get Their Asses Kissed," and "'Straight' Queer." These articles appeared alongside advice columns, interviews, parodies of mainstream news items, book reviews, and historical vignettes, making *Straight to Hell* a potent blend of what one reader called "'fantastic jerk-off material & consciousness raising stuff'" (5). Unlike most texts addressed either to "parents, police, teachers, judges, border guards and other moral guardians of heterosexual values" or to queers only inasmuch "as it tells them to clean up their act" (6), journals like *Straight to Hell, Heresies,* and *Fag Rag* pioneered a 'zine culture produced by and for queers. As Shively put it, "You are indeed in 'Dangerous Country' when you not only start listening to participants but even more begin cheering them on and participating yourself!"

(6). Working the boundaries between fact and fiction (Are these reports real? Does it matter?), between entitlement and marginalization, discipline and pleasure, such publications enacted the "sexual socialism" imagined by writers from Altman, Johnston, and Shively to Califia, Rubin, and Rechy.

Reading these documents of the sexual revolution today, we recognize how much we've lost not to death (many of these writers are still producing radical materials today) but to unremembering. The wit of titles such as "Watersports Is Baptism by a Buddy" has given way to an academic depressiveness. The materialist critique has ceded to psychosexual or discursive analyses removed from historical conditions. The call for collective and coalitional action has lost out to segregated appeals to specific identity categories (even while decrying the bankruptcy of identity politics) at conferences and journals geared to a niche audience. The emotional exuberance — the rage, amusement, passion, defiance, pride — has been replaced by negativity and "queer pessimism." A sense of humor has collapsed under the weight of theoretical rigor. More than any of these, however, what we have lost is the creative *certainty* that new and inventive sexways aren't just futural potentials but are being innovated everywhere, that the sexual revolution is not a hopeless daydream but is at hand. "Together we grow in consciousness," Hay assured us, "to generate issues, *and actions upon these issues,* which make manifest the fleshing out of our shared world-vision" (*Radically Gay,* 199). Or, as Shively succinctly stated, "We embody our dreams," urging, "Listen to us in motion, emotion" (*Meat,* 7–8).

Listen now, therefore, to writers who proclaimed that "our desires — to suck cock for instance — are creative, they are the road to creation, to the modification of reality" (Shively, "Indiscriminate Promiscuity," 263); that sex contains "life-enhancing, health-restoring qualities which make the risk of social and legal penalties worth taking" (Lipton, From *The Erotic Revolution,* 176–77), and that ours is "not only a revolution *against the traditional morality* but also a revolution *in favor of wholly new concepts of the function of sex* in society" (176); that liberation "entails not just freedom from sexual restraint, but also freedom for the fulfillment of human potential, a large part of which has been unnecessarily restricted by tradition, prejudice and the requirements of socialization" (Altman, "Liberation," 632); that sex is "'not simply a release but a *transformation* of

the libido: from sexuality constrained under genital supremacy to eroticization of the entire personality'" (Marcuse quoted in Altman, 635); that
"our difference is not created solely by oppression" but is "a preference, a
sexual preference" (Califia, "A Secret Side," 527); that liberation "does not
mean an end to struggle," but it does alter the ends for and the means by
which we struggle (Altman, "Liberation," 642). "We live loosely," as Shively
asserted: "we know nothing lasts," not because our psyches shatter while
sucking cock or grow melancholy in their reiterative self-alienation or
because we are doomed to depression, but "because there will always be
something more" (*Meat,* 7–8).

Queer theory, in contrast, has been cautious about invoking liberation,
or freedom, or struggle, or even transformation — all terms that have been
cast as reductive, naïve, outdated, tossed out with a discredited "identity politics." There are signs of hopeful change in this regard, as queer
theorists are starting to risk optimism, utopian longing, and historical
feelings. We want to believe that such work signals a post-post-traumatic
(re)turn in queer theory, of remembering rather than de-generational
forgetting. If so, then queer theory may again propose ways to resist what
Altman called "the desexualization of the concept of liberation" ("Liberation," 632). It will do so not by unremembering the past but by interpreting its achievements as well as its shortcomings, by understanding that
being visionary need not always mean looking forward but often requires
looking backward, like Lot's wife, at a Sodom that may turn out to be a
sexy place to live. We will need to renounce the model of progressive
time, as theorists of queer temporality have urged, and to understand
that in very real ways the past *is* our present, that as Rechy observed, by
engaging in "forbidden contacts" with "forbidden strangers," we might
well find "time crushed" (*The Sexual Outlaw,* 27), the past and future,
memory and aspiration, woven into a more pleasurable and equitable
present.

We live in different times and face some different circumstances than
did the sexual theorists of the 1960s and 1970s, most important the onset
of AIDS and the "online" revolution. Such changes make it impossible
and undesirable to re-create an earlier era exactly as it was. But if we challenge caricatures of the past as a time of uncritical essentialism, we might
rediscover theorists like Shively, who posited sexuality in opposition to all
concepts, including identity, conceived as "changeless, timeless, natural,

and as unavoidable or indefinite as death," a "fraud meant to prevent any questioning or change in the so-called 'reality'" ("Indiscriminate Promiscuity," 261). Looking to the past, we might recognize that only in a state of traumatic unremembering could gay men be reduced to "fatigue, ennui, boredom, ironic distancing, indirectness, arch dismissal, insincerity, and camp" or to patient puppets nodding in time to a liberation they thought was either in the future or without ongoing struggle. Looking to the past, we might see not only the theorists of the sexual revolution discussed here but also the early theorists of the AIDS epidemic, gay men and lesbians such as Douglas Crimp, Cindy Patton, Joseph Beam, Simon Watney, Samuel Delany, Gregg Bordowitz, Sarah Schulman, Paula Treichler, and David Wojnarowicz, who form a "time crush," with their predecessors, rather than a traumatic break in time. Looking to the past, we would find thinkers who called themselves "gay," "lesbian," "sex radicals," and, yes, even "queer," thinkers with an abundance of creativity, humor, good feeling, communitarianism, materiality, and willingness to risk *vision*. Without these, we cease being a force for change and become just another set of books on graduate school reading lists. Ours is emphatically not a call to abandon theory or give up on intellectual critique. But surely we are capable of more. After we sort through bad feelings, after we sever cruel attachments, after we are shattered by sex and our normality is troubled, *then* what? In answering that question, we may need to look elsewhere than to the horizon of the future. We may have to haunt the past rather than let it haunt us. We may have to sex the archive. Ultimately, we need more than memories. We need other lives, different values, and greater possibilities in the present. When memory serves, it helps us create these. The greatest obstacle to drawing inspiration from the past is not AIDS—the virus was never that powerful—but our own fears and anxieties, our own routine truisms, which, by making unremembering imperative, leave us in ashes rather than flame.

5. REMEMBERING A NEW QUEER POLITICS

Ideals in the Aftermath of Identity

Idealizing Loss

The previous chapter showed how appeals to the future risk unremembering the past. This chapter turns to the converse: how memories of loss sited in the past may become occasions for the invention of idealistic futures. We turn here to visual texts — art by Felix Gonzalez-Torres and Delmas Howe, Miguel Arteta's 2000 film *Chuck & Buck,* and Alexandra Juhasz's 2005 "Video Remains" — to analyze how ruminations on loss may become powerful means to articulate and defend particular social ideals. Our analysis places memory at the vanguard of a politics of ideality, a creative and forward-looking process that continues the social, political, and sexual idealizations that make the imaginative innovations of queer world-making possible.

Exemplifying the vital relationship between loss and idealism, Charley Shively, at the conclusion of his 1974 manifesto "Indiscriminate Promiscuity as an Act of Revolution," presented what at first appears a troubling paradox:

> I think this may be my own greatest fantasy and fear — that of loss and abandonment. I've always worried about loss, what happens when the

lover goes away, what if he leaves me, where then will I be. Such fear leads one to shut off, to be closed to loving, to protect oneself for fear of being wounded. And even coming to love the wound too deeply. Doubtless my own fantasy is my own particular one and cannot be exactly imposed on others, certainly not all faggots nor all society. Yet, I offer my humble solution, Indiscriminate Promiscuity, and wonder if it wouldn't allow for a society in which each person could be free to provide for themselves without dependency. (263)

That one might feel fear in the face of losing something or someone one loves, of experiencing a deep sense of abandonment and grief, and of accommodating oneself to that experience to the point of "loving the wound" is not surprising. What makes Shively's confession startling is how quickly he moves between loss and fantasy, even suggesting that loss leads to fantasy. What is gained from fantasizing loss? What *pleasures* attend the translation of fear into fantasy? One answer to these questions can be surmised from Shively's conclusion, which shifts from grievous loss to an idealistic vision of a free society of citizens made self-sufficient through indiscriminate promiscuity. For Shively, paradoxical as it may seem, loss does not derive from a utopian idealism that is necessarily fated to fail and therefore must lead to disheartening loss; rather, loss precedes and generates vision. This chapter explores that counterintuitive causality.

First, however, we want to foreground another paradox implied by the joining of loss and fantasy. To put it simply, loss implies experience, while fantasy implies the absence of that experience. Although Shively presumably experienced the pleasures he fears losing, the *ideal* that loss generates (of a free and self-sufficient society) has yet to be experienced. This is sensible enough, so long as loss and fantasy remain temporally distinct, one rooted in the past, the other in the future. What happens, though, when both are fused in the present, as they seem to be for Shively? When loss becomes simultaneous with fantasy, memory and idealism merge, suggesting that idealism may arise from traces of past experience, yes, but also that memory might arise from a projective imagination rather than from a recollected past. In other words, one need not have experienced an ideal in order to "remember" it or to craft memories that transmit and safeguard ideals. Or to quote Greta Garbo in the title role of the 1933 camp classic *Queen Christina*, "It is possible to feel nostalgia for a place one has never seen."[1] By the same token, if one conceives memory as a progressive and inventive articulation of yearning rather than as a naïve effort at transparent recuperation, one can feel nostalgia for a time through which one has not lived.

Memory unyoked from experience and reattached to imaginative idealism lies at the heart of Patrick Moore's 2004 study of gay life "before" and "after" AIDS. Moore contends, as we have, that shame over sexual memories of the past has led gay culture to a "dissociated assimilation that excludes all except those leading the most traditional of lives" (*Beyond Shame*, xxvii). Because shame "defines our view of a sexual past that segued into AIDS, confirming to us our worst fears about ourselves and lending the condemnation of bigots a truthful echo" (xxi–xxii), Moore argues, gay men mistakenly believe that if "there is no sex, no memory of sex, and no current sign of sexuality, then we can hope that AIDS will pass by our doorway this time" (xxvi). Refusing memory, gay men sacrifice sexuality "as the tool for radical change" (xxiv). Unlike those of us living today, Moore claims, gay men in the 1970s "used sex as the raw material for a social experiment so extreme" that he likens it to art (xxiv). To this call to remember in a conventional sense, Moore adds a complication: he didn't live through the sexual utopia of the 1970s. "My fascination with the sexual culture of the 1970s," Moore acknowledges, "derives largely from the fact that I did not experience it directly" (xxii). Having never experienced the 1970s does not prevent Moore from "remembering" it, however. "As a gay man who missed these years," he proclaims, "I refuse to abandon their memory" (xxv). The inaccessibility of "experience" as its grounds makes memory not transparent recovery but imaginative ideality.

We second Moore's call for inventive memory in the belief that such memory fills a need not met by firsthand recollection or archival research. As David Eng and David Kazanjian show in their deft interpretation of Walter Benjamin, conventional historiography is limited by an objective empiricism that memory (or, as Eng and Kazanjian prefer, melancholia) refutes. For Benjamin, historicism is "an encrypting of the past from a singular, empathic point of view: that of the victor," producing a failure of compassionate imagination he called "'indolence of the heart'" (in Eng and Kazanjian, *Loss*, 1–2). Seeking to close the past off from the present by claiming the end of struggle that connects the present to the past, invention to fact, historicism is, for Benjamin, the "'root cause of sadness'"

(2). Benjamin's insight proves especially important when we turn to the subject of sex and sexuality. Addressing both mainstream and marginalized historical subjects, conventional histories create methodological barriers to certain topics: affect, fantasy, desire, the nonmaterial forces that animate much public life for gays, lesbians, and queers. In the rare instances when historians address such topics, they treat them as content rather than as the basis for new methodologies (in which, for instance, one would read history from the perspective of desire or fantasy as opposed to producing histories *of* fantasy or desire).[2] Because queers are made the bearers of affect, whimsy, and desire, allowing heteronormativity (particularly masculinity) to be imagined in terms of reason, objectivity, and factuality, history told from a purported disinterested empirical perspective, even if it takes up queer life as its content, is necessarily told from a unqueer point of view. In calling narratives of pastness produced by queer "memories" rather than "histories," then, we do not intend to invoke firsthand experience but its opposite, imaginative potential — not transparent recuperation but reparative interpretation, not a lost experience or its attendant bad feelings ("sadness") but aspiration, not the perspective of the victor but the experience of those pushed to the margins for whom the outcome of struggle is still uncertain. Memory is not simply content, then; it is also, for us, a methodology, productive, we show in the sections that follow, of a community held together not by identity or even experience but by an idealism that, with Eng and Kazanjian, we conceive as "full of volatile potentiality and future militancies rather than as pathologically bereft and politically reactive" (5). Memory is thus the basis for what we call ideality politics.

While memory is creative and idealist, it often presents itself in narratives not of futural expectation ("utopianism") but of loss. The following section turns to Giorgio Agamben's *Stanzas: Word and Phantasm in Western Culture* for an account of the constitutive relationship between loss and idealism. In brief, we argue that loss is not the necessary outcome of idealism but rather a protective cover, guarding ideals from conventional dismissals of the utopian, the aspirational, and the fantasized as pie-in-the sky impracticality, impossible to manifest in the present and/or doomed to failure in the (not too distant) future. Idealistic proposals are often met with the assertion that since a particular ideal has never yet existed, it is fated never to exist, a logic of precedent related to our juridical understanding of civil possibility. Casting idealism into memory narratives of loss insists on the realizability of the ideal. If something has been lost, it must once have existed; if it has escaped our grasp, it once was held, however tenuously. Narratives of loss, then, countervene common dismissals of idealism and may therefore be effective statements not only of what *was* and has now been lost but (also) of what is yearned for and may still therefore be. This is the move "from trauma to prophesy" (Eng and Kazanjian, *Loss,* 10) that allows the past "to bear witness to the present," making memory "steadfastly alive for the political work of the present" (5–6). While Eng and Kazanjian understand this potential in relation to Freudian melancholia, we prefer Alexandra Juhasz's term "nostalgia" or, better yet, simply memory. We read the accounts of "remembered" loss discussed in this chapter, as signs not of vanquished pastness but of idealism, collective and inventive, only beginning to take shape.

The previous chapters examined the work of novelists, video- and filmmakers, architects, artists, and others who, like Moore, "remembered" a period they did not necessarily live through in order to articulate, like Shively, a connection between fear and fantasy, or, as we have revised this dyad, between loss and idealism. In the following sections, we demonstrate that memory narratives centered on loss are productive modes of social aspiration both for those who did not live through this loss and for those who did. Memories can be, as Juhasz observes of nostalgia, "a refiguring of time and feeling" that becomes "collective and also potentially productive of new feelings and knowledge that might lead to action" ("Video Remains," 321–22). To do so, memories must be perceived as windows onto social aspirations, as time warps that bring past and future into a viable present, collective, inventive, and transformative. Thus can memory serve as the basis of a persistent and progressive ideality politics.

Noonday Phantasms

The productive fusion of loss and idealism has a long history. They come together for Giorgio Agamben in his meditations on the medieval phenomenon of the Noonday Demon, which was believed to possess certain religious men with *acedia* or "sloth."[3] Agamben describes how those afflicted by the Noonday Demon lost interest in and became critical of the everyday practices of their cloistered lives (according to *De Octo Spiritibus*

Malitae, "the wretched one begins to complain that he obtains no benefit from conventional life" [in *Stanzas,* 4]), while simultaneously express-ing ecstatic praise for distant monasteries where they claimed they could find spiritual fulfillment (the slothful "plunges into exaggerated praise of distant and absent monasteries and evokes the places where he could be healthy and happy" within "pleasant communities of brothers" [in *Stanzas,* 4]). Unlike those who question or abandon divine good, those afflicted by the Noonday Demon preserved the ends, but not the approved means, of spiritual life, becoming in the process critical idealists. "What afflicts the slothful," Agamben writes, "is not therefore the awareness of an evil, but, on the contrary, the contemplation of the greatest of goods" (6).

Although *acedia* was initially characterized by what Agamben calls "the vertiginous and frightened withdrawal *(recessus)* when faced with the task implied by the place of man before God" (6), the slothful did not concede the ultimate unobtainability or incorporeality of their ideals. While the ideal status of divine truth safeguarded it from profanation, it also frustrated the capacity to embrace and embody that ideal. Caught between an idealizing inaccessibility and the desire to embrace, Agam-ben contends, those afflicted by the Noonday Demon manifested "*the perversion of a will that wants the object, but not the way that leads to it, and which simultaneously desires and bars the path to his or her own desire*" (6). The abyss opened "between desire and its unobtainable ob-ject" (6) could be bridged only by the creation of what Agamben calls *phantasms,* a mental image of an object that is both possessed (as an object of contemplative embrace) and idealized (protected from the loss and refusal imposed by anterior objects or people). Both corporeal and incorporeal, the phantasm paradoxically permits communication with the object of one's idealization "in the form of negation and lack" (7). Imagining "a world that is nearer to him than any other and from which depend, more directly than from physical nature, his happiness and his misfortune" (25), the slothful "open a space for the epiphany of the un-obtainable" and "testif[y] to the obscure wisdom according to which hope has been given only for the hopeless, goals only for those who will be unable to reach them" (7). Agamben's description of the phantasm as a visual image, at once recollected loss and projected fantasy, suggests why so many versions of idealist memory, including the ones discussed later in this chapter, take the form of art, video, and film.

Like those visual artists who turn repeatedly — and seemingly mournfully — to a history of loss, the religious men who were condemned as slothful came to be patients diagnosed as melancholic. But melancholy, in Agamben's account, is the reverse of Freud's psychic conservation. For Freud, melancholy preserves a lost object through psychic introjection, in which the bereaved, prevented by ambivalent feelings from detaching the libido from its lost object, incorporates its qualities into the self, thereby denying loss. This process, for Freud, is sadomasochistic, as the melancholic's hostility toward those qualities of the lost object that generated ambivalence is now directed toward the same qualities assumed as the melancholic's selfhood. While melancholy achieves a similar forestallment of loss for Agamben, he perceives the process not as a lost object without loss, as Freud did, but conversely as "a loss without a lost object" (20). For Agamben, melancholy cannot arise from a lost object, because the beloved, being ideal, has never been possessed and therefore cannot be lost. The "lost object," as a phantasm, in Agamben's counterintuitive inversion, is the creation of the melancholic psyche, generated to forestall loss. Melancholia as a projective fantasy thus "affects the paradox of an intention to mourn that precedes and anticipates the loss of the object," making viable "an appropriation in a situation in which none is really possible" (20). Unlike the slothful, whose phantasm of an ideal brotherhood could be dismissed as incorporeal and unobtainable, the supposedly lost object of melancholia bears traces of the real, of what once was and therefore might be again. Like the slothful, the melancholic creates a phantasm "at once real and unreal, incorporeal and lost, affirmed and denied" (21), but the melancholic's phantasm is triply protected: against the loss endemic to the unobtainable, against the corrupting handling of the conventional, and against the dismissive disregard suffered by the fantastic. Rather than a sadomasochistic process of self-abuse, melancholy becomes an imaginative process of projective psychic realization.

The ways that melancholy preserves the possibility of the fantastic are of particular interest to Agamben, for the fantastical and imaginary qualities of the phantasm make it a vehicle for progressive social change. The hope for change lies, in Agamben's analysis, in the unreal: in a realm of aspiration and untried options capable of posing critical alternatives to what the slothful criticized as "conventional life." Drawing material from the everyday but transforming it through the aspirational imagination, melancholy strategically "opens a space for the existence of the unreal and makes out a scene in which the ego may enter into relation with it and attempt an appropriation such as no other possession could rival and no loss possibly threaten" (20). Correcting a conventional world where "reality" is "narcissistically denied to the melancholic as an object of love, the phantasm yet receives from this negation a reality principle and emerges from the mute interior crypt in order to enter into a new and fundamental dimension," neither "the hallucinated oneiric scene of the phantasms nor the indifferent world of natural objects" (25).

Responsible "not only for the melancholics' morbid propensity for necromantic fascination but also for their aptitude for ecstatic illumination" (24), the phantasm, capable of challenging reality through "disjunction and excess" (17) while simultaneously granting trace reality to the unreal, becomes a powerful mode of progressive imagination. The traditional "affinity between melancholy and the imaginative faculty" (24) finds an explanation, for Agamben, in the former's phantasmatic invention, which is not only "the vehicle of dreams, of love, and of magical influence, but which also appears closely and enigmatically joined to the noblest creations of human culture" (25), a productive social imagination that is "constantly oriented in the light of utopia" (xix). Placing fantasy between love and desire, loss and projection, Agamben not only shows how melancholic ideality explains the transition from deprivation to vision so characteristic of queer creativity, he suggests as well the role in progressive imagination of eros and memory, which, by draping a desired object in the funereal garb of loss, manage to aspire toward and envision new desires, new socialities, new ideals.

While Agamben does not invoke sexual minorities, the relevance of his theorization of ideality politics bears striking affinities with gay and queer cultural politics. Among the groups most denied the fulfillments promised by conventional life, sexual minorities have made from that privation sensibilities both nostalgic and visionary. Our second chapter invoked camp as a particular deployment of nostalgia. Here we return to a more overtly erotic, gay sensibility discussed in chapter 1: Foucault's claim that "For a homosexual the best moment of love is likely to be when the lover leaves in the taxi," for it is only "when the act is over and the boy is gone that one begins to dream about the warmth of his body, the quality of his smile, the tone of his voice" ("Sexual Choice, Sexual

Act," 224). Memory, that is, allows for the creation of an ideal image (a "phantasm") that protects against the loss and disappointment that convention would seek to interject into the moment of love. Queer worldmaking similarly mixes memory and desire, shrouding ideals in the loss necessary to memory in order to assert that this once was and therefore might be again. The monks afflicted by the Noonday Demon, it bears remembering, not only withdrew from convention (as some antinormative queer theory has done) but moved *toward* "'pleasant communities of brothers'" (Agamben, *Stanzas*, 4). We might take such "pleasant communities" — comprising at once idealism and loss, invention and nostalgia, continually striving to reinvent codes of sociability in the face of deprivation and derision — as a phantasmatic ideal of sexual subculture. And if we ground such a subculture, as Agamben suggests, not on identity but on ideality, we can see why acts of gay memory are not normalizing attempts to reclaim transparently a necessarily (and, in some respects, gladly) lost past but an invitation to make loss and memory occasions to envision and protect new ideals.

If, as Agamben observes, "the libido behaves *as if* a loss has occurred even though *nothing* has in fact been lost, this is because the libido stages a simulation where what cannot be lost because it has never been possessed appears as lost, and what could never be possessed because it had never perhaps existed may be appropriated insofar as it is lost" (20). By claiming loss and memory as products and projections of idealization, we do not minimize devastating material losses or the suffering and grief occasioned by real deaths. But Agamben helps us reconsider the answers to important questions: Should we abandon memories because they cannot recapture a past that is irretrievably lost to us, or because they are idealizing? Is looking backward inimical to progressive politics? And, most important from our perspective, must traumatic loss necessarily naturalize a fallow period of cultural quietism rather than a resurgence of transformative and inventive idealism? The answer to these questions, in light of Agamben's analysis of memory's prophylactic phantasms, must be no.

We believe, with Douglas Crimp, that mourning is necessary to militancy, but so too is idealism, which motivates us to act on behalf not only of what has been and is threatened with loss but of what has not yet been but would make life more pleasurable, more equitable, more *ideal.*

The inaccessibility of the past is exactly why memory does creative and progressive work, for hope—what Agamben calls positivity—is available only through the unobtainability of the past. Creating ideal images to forestall losses that have not yet happened (the loss to homophobia and heteronormativity of radically inventive world-making rather than the material losses to AIDS, which can never be recovered), memory, as Agamben shows, replicates the structures of desire. To have memory, we might say, is to engage erotically with the past: to want to touch an object of critical investigation, keeping alive both the critical potential of meditation and the utopian hope that an ideal may still be realized. This is why we cannot afford to live without memory, any more than we can live without hope, especially in the face of material losses that remain beyond the power of recollection to reclaim. Agamben notes, tellingly in the language of fatal epidemiology, "As of a mortal illness containing in itself the possibility of its own cure, it can be said of *acedia* that 'the greatest disgrace is never to have had it'" (7).

Visualizing Loss

AIDS became, Simon Watney attests, "a crisis of memory," a crisis registered by the difficulty of creating and sustaining adequate memorialization. When the deaths of loved ones "are casually dismissed as 'self-inflicted,'" Watney writes, "it is the most fundamental level of our most intense experience of life and of love that is effectively denied" (*Imagine Hope,* 156). At the same time, not all acts of memorialization do justice to the losses they mark, and Watney warns against "the types of pretentiously over-intellectualized justifications for politically correct 'invisible monuments,' or equally over-aestheticized 'self-destructing memorials' which in effect merely collude with the very processes of selective historical amnesia that effective memorial art is intended to arrest, or at least delay" (152). Much of the difficulty in memorializing the losses due to AIDS lies in finding a balance between an aesthetic appeal that draws viewers to contemplate the experience of loss and one that diverts attention from the materiality of loss, between a monument that captures a sense of time and one that deadens time into a transcendent abstraction. The phrase "Imagine Hope," the title of Watney's collection of essays on AIDS representation, is drawn from a cover illustration for the "Gay Life

'89" special issue of the *Village Voice* (262) and alludes to the need for visual representation, for images, equal to our needs. We need memorials that are iconic and intangible, inspiring both an experience of loss and a determination to survive and to change the historical conditions that made loss possible and then, adding insult to injury, made it forgettable. The difficulty comes, in other words, in finding an aesthetic balance between loss and hope or idealism (for what hope is possible without a yearned-for ideal?).

Gay culture has struggled to strike this balance. Writing in 1994, Watney cited "monuments to our loved ones everywhere from quilts to personal altars in the picture windows of community shops, to gardens" (*Imagine Hope*, 163). These vernacular memorials sprang up in response to the urgent need to commemorate individuals. In their proliferation in certain sites — neighborhoods and street protests, for example — their multiplicity also constituted, in Watney's words, "a highly creative, constantly changing collective memorial" (163). As the populations recognized as affected by AIDS changed, the nature and meaning of AIDS memorials, quite appropriately, changed too. The NAMES Project Quilt, to which Watney alluded in his list of vernacular monuments, is a case in point. The Quilt, conceived in 1985 during a march commemorating the assassination of Harvey Milk, was first realized as a forty-panel memorial to be hung from San Francisco's City Hall during the Lesbian and Gay Freedom Parade in June 1987. By October of that year, when it was displayed in Washington, D.C., during the National March for Gay and Lesbian Rights, it included almost two thousand three-by-six foot fabric panels.[4] The Quilt's origins in the political activism of the San Francisco gay community was reflected in the location in the Castro of the NAMES Project's first storefront office, as well as in the "wish list" for donated materials posted outside that office — it requires a collective sensibility steeped in camp to imagine a memorial to the dead appropriately created of "sequins, beads, fabric, and glue" (Ruskin, *The Quilt*, 9). As the demographics of AIDS activism expanded beyond the gay community, however, and the Quilt grew to commemorate, by one recent count, over 82,000 dead, its function as a memorial to gay culture ceded to its status as "the epidemic's . . . most national memorial," as analyzed by Marita Sturken in the context of other national memorials such as the Vietnam War Memorial (*Tangled Memories*, 183). As Sturken notes, "Debates about

how 'gay' the quilt is, and its relationship to the gay community" arose
by 1988 and remained "central to its meaning" (206, 211). More conventional AIDS memorials in North American cities from Vancouver to
Key West — which share a stony monumentality, repeated rectilinear elements, and lists of inscribed names — adopted the visual rhetoric of the
war memorial, casting the deaths inflicted by AIDS as losses to the *polis,*
specifically to the city in which the monuments are sited but more generally to the nation. Without wishing in any way to stigmatize either the
inclusion of nongay victims of AIDS in AIDS memorials or the concep-
tualization of the loss of these gay and nongay people as losses to their
cities and states, it is important to acknowledge that these types of visual
memorialization of AIDS inadequately fill the need for the memorialization of the gay culture(s) lost as a result of the AIDS crisis.

We should not expect that collectively created memorials to individuals lost to AIDS will, as a side effect, memorialize gay culture. Such efforts, heartfelt and moving as they are, will be subsumed into civic or
national identities or be lost to their own ephemerality, falling into a
vacuum of unremembering and miscomprehension. Even the largest and
most various of the AIDS memorials, the NAMES Project Quilt — its individual panels recording a touching and exhilarating fusion of political
energy, subcultural affirmation, and articulations of nonnational forms
of connection, especially mother-love — has not escaped these fates. Repeatedly displayed on the National Mall in Washington, it has in recent
years almost disappeared from view, ambitious plans for its permanent
display indefinitely postponed.

What is needed now is an aesthetics of memory that can articulate the
relationship of loss and hope, of commemoration and idealism in relation to gay culture — memorials that will help us to overcome our traumatized forgetfulness of the gay past. As important as commemorating
the past, these memorials (and memory narratives more generally) must
renovate the past in light of our present ideals, inviting viewers to create
inventive hybrids of a past loss that will move us from our contemporary unremembering into a current idealism that will turn the past into a
more just and satisfying present.

Just such an aesthetics of memory and memorialization can be found
in the work of Cuban American visual artist Felix Gonzalez-Torres, whose
candy spills, paper stacks, posters, and installations compose a phantas-

matic memorialization that achieves both commemoration and idealism.[5] Gonzalez-Torres located his aesthetic motivation in despair over
contemporary unremembering. In the early 1990s, explaining that his
experience as a teacher showed him that "kids had no historical reference" and "the Republican Party's biggest voting block is kids below thirty,"
Gonzalez-Torres concluded: "The only people who learned anything in
the 60s were on the [political] right" (in Nickas, "Felix Gonzalez-Torres,"
87). Against this forgetting, Gonzalez-Torres made art as "an attempt to
create a kind of historical picture, a reminder, to reinstate certain events"
and to allow "people to project themselves into those events" (87). Generating combinations of projections and recollections, Gonzalez-Torres's
art allows viewers to experience the past, with all the attendant experiences of loss, while maintaining their *presentness*. From the interface between past and present comes his art's potential for critique and idealism,
each moment in time showing but also supplementing the limitations of
the other.

Gonzalez-Torres's art shows how intrinsically the movement from
spectatorship to speculation, from vision to visionary, relies on the elision of temporal succession and its fictions of progress. Writing on the
back of a photograph, Gonzalez-Torres posed the question, "Can we take
a second for granted?" and answered:

> Never. Never. A second is all it takes for life to dissipate. And, what do
> you see? An empty room. But not really. We see history: light, noise,
> smell, beginnings, dinners, soft long mornings, play, laughter, phone
> rings, some tears, hope, sex and love, excitement, sadness, history his-
> tory history. (in Moore, *Beyond Shame*, 170)

Faced with loss, with life dissipated, Gonzalez-Torres produced vision,
first literal ("What do you see?"), but then more metaphysical, more *visionary*. Significantly, the shift from loss to vision takes place at the site not
of utopian projection but of history: backward looking, reminiscent, at
once intimate and social. In locating an intimate ideal — "tears, hope, sex
and love" — as an always-already lost "history," Gonzalez-Torres grounded
his aesthetic vision in the combination of prophylactic loss and projective idealism that Agamben calls *acedia*. Having been lost, the intimate
ideal Gonzalez-Torres evoked must have existed at one time, must have
once been possessed. Thus his vision sheds its status *as* ideal, becoming

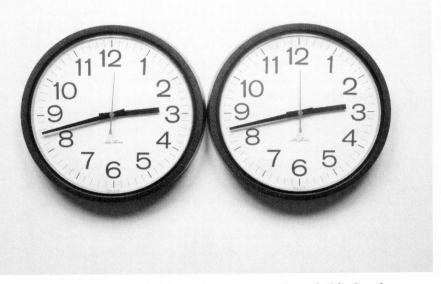

Felix Gonzalez-Torres, *"Untitled" (Perfect Lovers)*, 1987–90. Copyright Felix Gonzalez-Torres Foundation. Courtesy of Andrea Rosen Gallery, New York.

something more corporeal, more tangible, and more *possible*. And yet, contemplated only in the mind's eye (vision in the second sense), the ideal is projective, irreducible to the imperatives of the already-tried and the disappointments of loss or failed attainment.

Possible and lost, corporeal and imminent, Gonzalez-Torres's vision is very close to how one might characterize desire—or describe identity. This proximity is not surprising. The ideal Gonzalez-Torres aestheticized incorporates both the longing for identity that persists as a communal ideal and the perpetual unsettling of that ideal by the longings that disrupt and keep potentially in process a sense of collective belonging. Finding a rare balance between identity and desire, Gonzalez-Torres's *acedia* may become the basis for a transformative queer politics of the ideal.

Gonzalez-Torres's art is saturated by loss, both personal (the death from AIDS of his lover Ross Laycock and his own diagnosis with HIV)

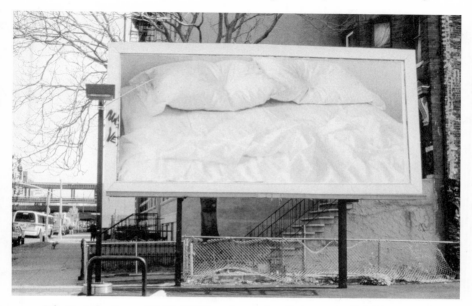

Felix Gonzalez-Torres, *"Untitled,"* billboard, 1991. Installation at 2511 Third Avenue, Bronx, for *Projects 34: Felix Gonzalez-Torres* at the Museum of Modern Art, New York, 1992. Copyright Felix Gonzalez-Torres Foundation. Courtesy of Andrea Rosen Gallery, New York.

and collective (the artist described watching as "a whole generation be-comes a flock of birds, flying away, traveling, gone to an unexplained place" while "we, in shock," watch from below [in Moore, *Beyond Shame*, 170]). Works such as *"Untitled" (Perfect Lovers),* in which two identical clocks tick away side by side in perfect unison until inevitably the bat-teries of one wear down and, falling behind its mate, it eventually stops altogether, or his 1991 billboard depicting an empty bed still bearing the imprint of bodies no longer present, signify a quotidian loss connected to "a fear of losing everything" (in Spector, *Felix Gonzalez-Torres,* 122). The loss depicted in the work is both personal and public, and its depic-tion evokes both historical record and individual memory.

As the clocks suggest, time is central to Gonzalez-Torres's work. Even pieces that don't refer directly to time — the stacks of identical papers or the spills of candy, both of which invite viewers to take away pieces of the sculpture as souvenirs, only to be replenished periodically — create a

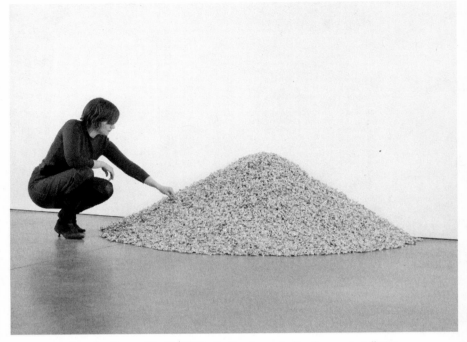

Felix Gonzalez-Torres, *"Untitled" (Placebo-Landscape for Roni)*, 1993. Installation at *Felix Gonzalez-Torres and Roni Horn* at Andrea Rosen Gallery, New York, 2001. Copyright Felix Gonzalez-Torres Foundation. Courtesy of Andrea Rosen Gallery, New York.

seriality that introduces time into the aesthetic process. Gonzalez-Torres said that the experience of watching his sculptures drift away piece by piece — "a very masochistic practice" — prepared him for larger, more inevitable losses. "This work is about controlling my own fears. My work cannot be destroyed. I have destroyed it already, from day one," Gonzalez-Torres explained, adding, "This work cannot disappear. This work cannot be destroyed the way other things in my life have disappeared and have left me. I destroyed it myself instead. I had control over it and this is what empowered me" (122).

If Gonzalez-Torres's art making invokes masochistic loss, it also involves a preservation. He says of his works, "They will always exist because they don't really exist, or because they don't have to exist all the time" (in Bartman et al., *Between Artists*, 94). This balance between loss and preservation pivots on the translation of material bodies (which can be "lost" both to time and to their own autonomy) into ideal images (the paper stacks are replenished to an ideal height, the candy spills to an ideal weight) that resemble what Agamben describes as the medieval phantasm. More than simple testimonies of loss, the sculptures are aesthetic acts of *acedia*. Flouting conventional imperatives toward useful work in their passivity and generosity (museum visitors often express anxiety about helping themselves to the elements that are there for the taking in the art), Gonzalez-Torres's "sloth" reveals itself as a socially intimate ideal persistently generated across and *against* a seemingly imperative temporality.

Gonzalez-Torres linked his ideas to the German poet Rainer Maria Rilke, who articulated the transformation of memory from an archive of loss to a seedbed of inventive idealization. In order to create, Rilke claimed, one must "have memories of many nights of love, one must also have been beside the dying, must have sat beside the dead in the room with the open window." And yet, Rilke acknowledged, "it is not yet enough to have memories. For it is not yet the memories themselves." Rather, memories must "have turned to blood within us, to glance and to gesture, nameless and no longer to be distinguished from ourselves" and only then "can it happen that in the most rare hour the first word of a verse arises in their midst and goes forth from there" (in Spector, *Felix Gonzalez-Torres*, 42). As Nancy Spector notes, Gonzalez-Torres took from Rilke the desire to combine intimate "blood memories" with collective public history to generate "a multivalent narrative in which the intimate and the communal are fused" (54). This fusion is related to the awareness — also present in Rilke — that memory is not a transparent re-creation of the past but an imaginative combination of criticism and invention that allows us to wrestle ideals from the losses of the past in order to contemplate them, imaginatively, as possibilities in the present and options for the future.

This mixing of past and present, of loss and idealism, had particular implications for queer cultural politics, especially in the face of AIDS. "I do have a political and personal agenda with this work, and in a way they are very interrelated," Gonzalez-Torres claimed (in Bartman et al.,

Between Artists, 96), and Roland Wäspe has recognized the way his blurring of categories of public in private is linked to the artist's response to the 1986 Supreme Court decision affirming "that gay men and lesbian women have no right to a private sphere, because the state . . . can invade their bedrooms to check and punish them" ("Private and Public," 18). A small 1987 Photostat "portrait" consists of a reflective black background along the bottom of which run white lines of text reading, "supreme 1986 court crash stock market crash 1929 sodomy stock market court stock supreme 1987" (Elger, "Catalogue Raisonné," 25).[6] Collapsing present and past, this personal rearrangement of terms from public discourse suggests a commensurate sense of "crash" in the financial and erotic realms. A room-scale self-portrait—also from 1987 and also consisting of lines of text, though these words are painted around the walls of a gallery at ceiling level—included "Stonewall 1969" among the significant dates (Wäspe, "Private and Public," 19), although the artist was only ten years old and living in Puerto Rico at that time.

Combining history and memory, loss and replenishment, his work represents Gonzalez-Torres's ideal projection of gay culture into a future made uncertain by AIDS and its debilitating losses. "With the stack pieces," critic Robert Nickas observes, "you can take a rolled up sheet from the gallery and 'get the piece,' but there's no way you can remove it entirely. It's portable, yet unmovable" ("Felix Gonzalez-Torres," 88). When Gonzalez-Torres, responding to Nickas, concurs, "We are everywhere, we will always be here no matter what they do" (88), he echoes the popular gay liberation slogan ("We are everywhere"), now taken from the past and turned into a defiant ideal of future-oriented invincibility. When the artist claimed his work "cannot be destroyed," it is not just because, as he says, he has always already destroyed it, but because he has moved from the empirically visual to a visionary ideal, protecting his politics of ideality, counterintuitively, in the melancholy guise of fear, anxiety, and loss. Adapting the seemingly free-associated lists from his small-scale (around 8 by 10 inches) Photostat and room-scale text portraits, Gonzalez-Torres in 1989 installed a billboard above Sheridan Square (near the site of the Stonewall riots) listing, in white type against a black background, historical events that might be said to define a collective gay consciousness:

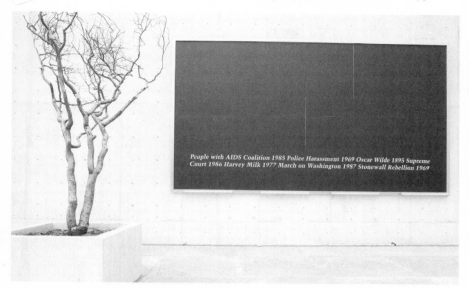

People with AIDS Coalition 1985 Police Harassment 1969 Oscar Wilde 1895 Supreme Court 1986 Harvey Milk 1977 March on Washington 1987 Stonewall Rebellion 1969

Felix Gonzalez-Torres, *"Untitled,"* billboard, 1989. Installation at *Somewhere/Nowhere* at Museo Universitario Arte Contemporáneo, Mexico City, 2010. Copyright Felix Gonzalez-Torres Foundation. Courtesy of Andrea Rosen Gallery, New York.

People With AIDS Coalition 1985 Police Harassment 1969 Oscar Wilde 1895 Supreme Court 1986 Harvey Milk 1977 March on Washington 1987 Stonewall Rebellion 1969

The links between personal history and community history are clear in the way the 1987 room-scale self-portrait described above intermixes some of these events ("Supreme Court 1986 March on Washington 1987") with more autobiographical references ("Venice 1985 Paris 1985"), and adds the instruction, as a requirement of ownership, that the curators gradually replace the items from the artist's list with items of their own — the curators at the Art Institute of Chicago recently added "Election Night Grant Park 2008."[7]

Combining defeat and hopefulness — assassinations and juridical setbacks alongside marches and rebellions — this art emphasizes the connection between loss and idealism that runs throughout Gonzalez-Torres's oeuvre. Just as important, however, is the artist's disordering of chronology, suggesting, as Watney observes, that history is not "a seamless progressive narrative, expressing some supposedly unified historical force or will. Rather, events and institutions coexist, as in memory, in no particular order or sequence beyond that of our own active interpretive making. The 'private' defiantly invades 'public' space" (*Imagine Hope*, 158). It is this transformation of history into memory that allows contemporary viewers to feel a part of events they may or may not have lived through, to commemorate as part of living sensation, and to deny the pastness of history by turning it into a vision of possibility for the present and future.

A similar process becomes evident in one of Gonzalez-Torres's most complex pieces, the 1991 installation titled *Every Week There Is Something Different*, which evolved sequentially over three weeks. The first week featured a display of photographs of thirteen words inscribed around the base of the Theodore Roosevelt memorial at New York's Museum of Natural History. In the second week, Gonzalez-Torres removed all but three of the photographed inscriptions — "Soldier," "Humanitarian," "Explorer" — and built in the center of the gallery a blue platform outlined with large lightbulbs. During the third week, a go-go dancer, naked except for silver briefs, tennis shoes, and a walkman, danced at intervals on the platform. This seemingly whimsical piece has serious implications. The culture represented by go-go dancing — discos, bars, sex clubs — was by 1991 in Manhattan itself a kind of endangered species, though not of the sort displayed in the Museum of Natural History. Gonzalez-Torres shifts the rhetorics of loss and memorialization, replacing the fossilized time of the Roosevelt monument (and, for that matter, the Natural History Museum) with the living unpredictable time of go-go dancing, the imperial figure of Roosevelt with the erotic figure of the dancer, the aesthetic distance and social propriety associated with the art gallery with the awkward yet enthralling immediacy of a living exhibitionist, with all the conflicting connotations of deviant pleasure and exploitation that go-go dancing arouses. Although eroticism and sex culture are rarely the stuff of conventional memorials, the three photographed words that Gonzalez-Torres left hanging behind the go-go dancer — soldier, humanitarian, and explorer — inscribe this living "monument" with the attributes of courage, compassion, and curious exploration. These virtues borrowed from the monumentalized past assert the worth of marginalized sex cultures defined, now, less in terms of space (moving the dancer into

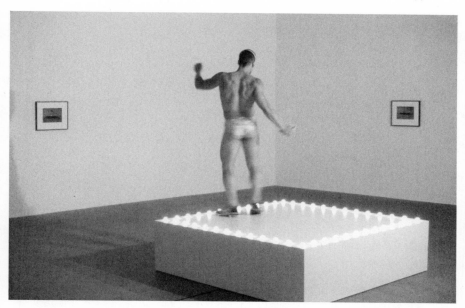

Felix Gonzalez-Torres, *"Untitled" (Go-Go Dancing Platform)*, 1991. Installation at *Every Week There Is Something Different*, Andrea Rosen Gallery, New York, 1991. Photograph by Peter Muscato. Copyright Felix Gonzalez-Torres Foundation. Courtesy of Andrea Rosen Gallery, New York.

the gallery fails to queer the space through performance but rather emphasizes the vulnerability of both the dancer and the dance) than of the dynamics of time, both remembered and anticipated. *"Untitled" (Go-Go Dancing Platform)* combines what Gonzalez-Torres described as the "fear of loss and the joy of living, of growing, changing, of always becoming more, of losing oneself slowly and then being replenished all over again from scratch" (in Bartman et al., *Between Artists*, 95).

Gonzalez-Torres's other sculptures similarly engage issues of loss and renewal, danger, desire, and hope. The sculptures he called "light strings" literally radiate a warm glow, a light that can read as enlightenment and/or hope (the proverbial light at the end of the tunnel) — or as the fusion of those affects that is optimism. The first of these works in 1991 comprised a set of single bulbs, each on its own extension cord (Elger, "Catalogue Raisonné," 69), but the light pieces quickly became strings of lights and then groups of strings of lights. Sometimes — as in *Lovers-Paris* — these

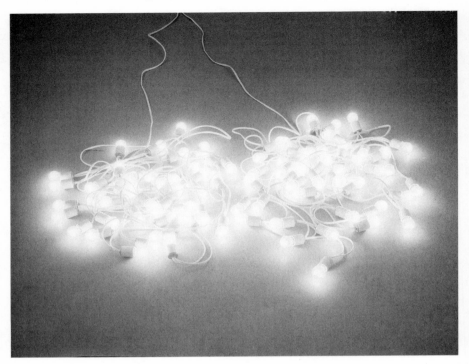

Felix Gonzalez-Torres, *"Untitled" (Lovers–Paris),* 1993. Copyright Felix Gonzalez-Torres Foundation. Courtesy of Andrea Rosen Gallery, New York.

were titled in ways that encouraged anthropomorphic readings. Two hanging strands subtitled *Couple* adorned the cover of *Melancholia and Moralism,* Douglas Crimp's important book theorizing the relationship of loss to AIDS activism. Allusions to private meanings rooted in memory here fuse with a collective aesthetic suggested by the multiplicity of lights. Collectivity becomes an ideal — a phantasm — that guards against loss: one or two bulbs may burn out and be disposed, but the collective light, shared but belonging to no single source, continues. The only requirement for the installation of the light strings, according to the artist, is that, when they are illuminated, all the bulbs must be lit.

Gonzalez-Torres's candy sculptures also incorporate an ideal of collective public pleasure that works dialectically with the cycles of loss. Inviting viewers to take pieces of candy, Gonzalez-Torres invokes his audiences' desires and pleasures — the sensual pleasures of sucking (especially, when he subtitles the sculpture *Portrait of Ross in L.A.*, of sucking on his lover's body), the energy released by sugar, the ephemeral and slightly guilty connection with anonymous others taking part in a collective and public experience of endlessly available pleasure, the refusal to heed childhood warnings never to accept candy from strangers—that the passage of time cannot eradicate. "I'm giving you this sugary thing," Gonzalez-Torres said; "you put it in your mouth and you suck on someone else's body. And in this way, my work becomes part of so many other people's bodies. It's very hot" (in Spector, *Felix Gonzalez-Torres*, 147–50). Creating what Nancy Spector calls "pliant, savory bodies languorously waiting to be plucked and consumed" (147), Gonzalez-Torres gives us an experience both lost and always keenly anticipated, achingly personal, and comprising, in his words, "one enormous collaboration with the public" in which the "pieces just disperse themselves like a virus that goes to many different places—homes, studios, shops, bathrooms, wherever" (58). If his viral analogy invokes the anxious losses caused by AIDS, it also reminds us of the persistence and ingenuity of ideals, which make their way, like the candies, into places both personal and public.

These sculptures are not without their edge, for ideals invariably give rise to dissenting critique (just as critiques always imply a persistent ideal). How can you blame me for deciding to suck, despite the risk, the artist seems to ask, when you decided to suck as well, despite not knowing if the candy is tainted? How do you decide whom to trust? When Gonzalez-Torres calls the piece made from black licorice *Public Opinion* or one made from Bazooka bubble gum *Welcome Back Heroes* (both 1991), the art poses sharper questions: Are you free from the desire for which you judge others, or are your desires for conformity of opinion, xenophobic self-satisfaction, or military mass destruction all more addictive and dangerous than the pleasures you would condemn? As Gonzalez-Torres observed, his *USA Today* spill (1990) made from red, white, and blue suckers was "a 'sugar rush.' With patriotism you get really high, very euphoric. But then you come down" (in Nickas, "Felix Gonzalez-Torres," 89). The piece *"Untitled" (Placebo)* (1990), made from over one thousand pounds of silver-wrapped candy, invokes the "double-blind" testing process of the medical research that gave people with AIDS [PWAs] sugar pills in place of life-saving medications. The needs of PWAs seem again on Gonzalez-Torres's mind in the 1991 *"Untitled" (Blue Cross)*, in which

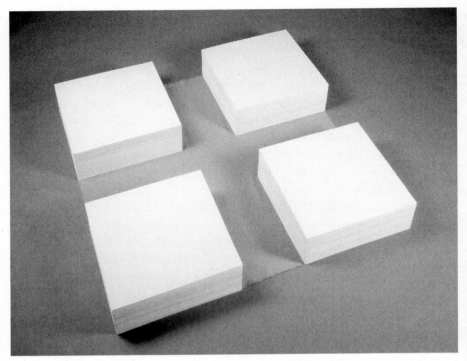

Felix Gonzalez-Torres, *"Untitled" (Blue Cross)*, 1990. Photograph by Peter Muscato. Copyright Felix Gonzalez-Torres Foundation. Courtesy of Andrea Rosen Gallery, New York.

the paper stack brings to mind the endless paperwork involved in claiming insurance benefits.

Although "in its excessive generosity—its willingness to give itself away to any admiring beholder"—Gonzalez-Torres's art "risks the danger of total dissipation," as Spector puts it (*Felix Gonzalez-Torres,* 154), his corpus of work persistently moves, as Spector also acknowledges, "from memory to fantasy" (62). A similar trajectory characterizes the very different work of another contemporary artist, Delmas Howe. Howe's life and work were centered in the burgeoning New York gay community in the 1960s and 1970s, where he made a name for himself with paintings that pictured Greco-Roman myth with a cast of cowboys in the settings of his native New Mexico. After he returned to his hometown of Truth or Consequences and his partner died from AIDS in 1993, Howe's paintings

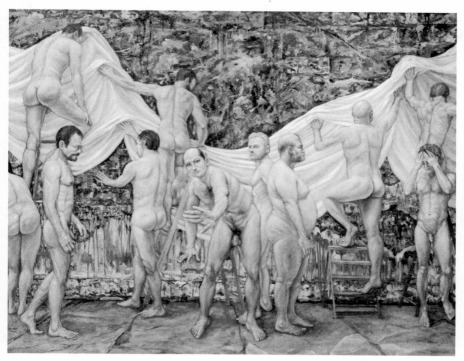

Delmas Howe, *Wall III: Survivors,* 2008. Photograph courtesy of Delmas Howe and RioBravoFineArt, Inc., Truth or Consequences, New Mexico.

began to take on Biblical themes, now set in spaces drawn from his memories of what he calls the "sexual theatre" of the West Side piers during the 1970s (discussed in chapter 2).[8] "The paintings," Howe has stated, "are intended to evoke a conglomeration of feelings: the celebration of sexuality and the male body that the sex piers represented, the thrill of all that sex so openly available at the time, and of course the grief that has followed with AIDS" (Strong, "Coloring the World Queer"). The paintings in Howe's recent *Gray Wall Series* return directly to these themes. *Wall III: Survivors* (from which our cover illustration for this book is taken) depicts eleven naked men of different body types and ages endeavoring to cover a black and decaying wall with what Howe calls "the white cloth of hope."[9] The painting conveys the efforts of "survivors" (of homophobia, of AIDS) who endeavor to cover their bleak backdrop with something more fluid, more possible, more ideal. The work of survival necessitates such efforts, even as the scarred bleakness of the wall, suggesting the losses experienced by gay men, makes visible the hopeful endeavor represented by the cloth. Here "survival" is undertaken collectively, as in Gonzalez-Torres's light pieces, and the large format of the four-by-six-foot canvas gives that collective idealism a monumental feel. Perhaps this is the kind of monument, no longer ephemeral or co-optable, that Watney imagined as a proper commemoration of the losses and ideals that have sustained gay men *as* a culture. For Gonzalez-Torres as for Howe, the cycle of memory and fantasy, of loss and optimism, when turned into an aesthetics of *acedia*, not only forestalls loss through commemorative memory, it imagines, on the pretext of loss, new collectives, new oppositions, new ideals as the ongoing art/work of gay men's lives after AIDS.

Bucking Loss

Unlike Felix Gonzalez-Torres, Buck O'Brien is not the sort of artist whose work is ever going to disrupt the protocols of the museum. For starters, he is a fictional character in the 2000 film *Chuck & Buck,* and in the plot of the film, his art is not intended for the galleries but for an audience of one: his childhood friend Charlie "Chuck" Sitter (Chuck is indeed Buck's only "sitter" for his art). The dynamics of art-making and art-viewing in the film resonate with our analysis of Gonzalez-Torres, however, in their shared deployment of the past to collapse fictions of progressive temporality and thus to critique normative institutions and to introduce, in the guise of loss, ideals of intimate generosity that far exceed the possibilities permitted by what Lauren Berlant calls "major intimacies," that is, those with institutional sanction.[10] Observing that Gonzalez-Torres's art conjures images of "childhood, games, and play" through its invocation of "memory rooted in childhood," critic Robert Nickas foregrounds the critical alternative posed by this childlike idealism: "There is," he writes, "a free relationship to the world which lasts very briefly in our lives before rules and biases are set, and we are captive to specific patterns of behavior" ("Felix Gonzalez-Torres," 86). *Chuck & Buck* takes up that potential, examining what it might look like if adult "rules and biases" failed to quash childhood ideals. Minor intimacies, Berlant observes, often require an extreme aesthetic, and the film, repeatedly characterized by critics as "creepy," exaggerates the explosive queerness of infantile memory.[11]

Perhaps the queerest film of its day, *Chuck & Buck* thus offers a powerful alternative to imperatives that insist that gay men, through unremembering, overcome the play (sexual and otherwise) of our (cultural) youth and become "mature," if significantly less happy, adults. Played by Mike White, who also wrote the screenplay, Buck refuses to grow up into "mature" heteronormativity. Instead, the persistently infantile Buck makes his memories, never free from sadness and loss, into a powerful source of social idealism that, however mocked and pathologized, allows him, through the temporal displacements of memory, to buck loss and achieve a more fulfilling collective life in the here and now.

At the film's start, twenty-two-year-old Buck seems the classic subject of a dozen made-for-television melodramas, if not to say Freudian case histories. *Chuck & Buck* opens with a traumatic event: as the camera pans through a series of close-ups of windup toys, plastic soldiers, and other childhood paraphernalia, we eventually focus not on the child we might expect but on a young man sucking a lollipop as he folds his laundry. As the sequence continues, we hear increasingly frantic coughing in the next room, where, we soon learn, Buck's mother is dying. The mise-en-scène, hovering unstably between *Psycho* and an afterschool special, suggests the crisis of the film will center on the man-child's loss of his sole source of care. More darkly, the opening suggests a classic homophobic narrative (again, think of *Psycho*) in which a boy's attachment to his (distant and ultimately abandoning) mother leads to arrested development in the traumatized and desexualized son.

The opening of *Chuck & Buck* is a visual tease, however, for the film's soundtrack soon introduces a campy counternarrative in the form of Gwendolyn and the Good Time Gang's sing-songy tune "Freedom of the Heart," which cheerfully proclaims, "I got freedom of the heart / It's a brand new start / I see the sun shining through the trees in the park / ooodily ooodily ooodily oodily oodily oodily fun fun fun." This juxtaposition of loss and possibility, crisis and freedom, signals the film's deployment of memory as an intervention in the normative assumptions hinted at by the film's opening: that a nostalgic adherence to childhood signifies arrested development and hence helplessness, that location within a conventional home suggests that familial ties are the primary source of support and emotional investment, that death signifies irredeemable loss, that childhood and eroticism are mutually exclusive except insofar as a child is the victim of adult sexual predation. Such assumptions are undermined by the ever-resilient Buck, who, far from being a grief-stricken and helpless innocent, is, it turns out, a man with a mission.

Buck has an erotic fixation on his childhood friend Chuck, now a Los Angeles music executive with a live-in fiancée. Although Buck has not seen Chuck since the latter's family moved away when the boys were eight, Buck has kept his photos of Chuck as pristine as his aspiration for an eventual reunion, for which his mother's death becomes a convenient occasion. Buck invites Chuck to the funeral and, in a scene critics have found among the film's most disturbing, watches the chapel door until Chuck enters, at which point the beaming Buck begins waving like an excited child. Further defying propriety, Buck ignores Chuck's introduction of his fiancée, Carlyn, focusing exclusively on his long-lost friend. "I'm glad you could make it, you know," he tells Chuck, "I think about you all the time. Us as kids and stuff." When Chuck, startled, attempts to restore polite convention by telling Buck, "You don't look much different," Buck responds, "You do. Your face is fatter." In spite of himself, Chuck laughs, the only time in the film he seems genuinely tickled. Chuck's amusement marks a rupture in the conventions attending memory. Whereas Chuck's conception of static memory seeks to establish temporal and intimate distance (Buck doesn't look "that different" only if Chuck neither remembers what Buck looked like as a child nor has looked closely at that child's current manifestation), Buck, although seemingly more invested in a recovered past, nevertheless acknowledges that time changes memory and the subjects it constitutes. Memory, for Buck, is not recuperation but a form of interpersonal engagement in the here and now animated by his creative response to differences between past and present.

A good deal is at stake in this exchange. Normative heterosexuality relies on a double disavowal that Judith Butler calls its "never-never" status.[12] Denying a primary erotic cathexis on a same-sex parent, according to Butler, the "mature" adult must also deny the grief occasioned by that disavowal. For Butler, therefore, heterosexuality is queer melancholy, as the "mature" heterosexual takes out on himself or herself (through shameful grief) the disavowed erotic pleasure once taken in the parent's body. We might make Butler's queer analysis even queerer, however, if we take the denied cathexis to be not familial but social, involving not a father but a friend (Freud, after all, says that melancholy may arise from the loss of a "near neighbor").[13] In that case, the disavowal necessary to "mature" heterosexuality would not produce psychic absence (a queer ontology) but the social crisis of loss. If rendering loss as absence naturalizes the operations of psychic disavowal and hence of agency (does one have control over one's infantile cathexis?) *as* heterosexuality, returning absence to loss restores the agency-granting possibility of social plenitude *as* queerness. If the second disavowal is not *necessary* to psychic development (if we don't *need* to disavow loss, transforming it into self-abusing absence), if the sociopsychic trajectory of "maturation" can be rerouted by traumatic disruption, we might retain the possibility, by restoring to some degree the lost social object, of a frustrated, if not entirely "cured," melancholy. Loss might become, in short, a call to nonnormative sociality, to community formation, to ideality politics.

Illustrating this possibility, Chuck's "normal" lifestyle in the film seems to consist of an exhaustingly continuous round of repressing not his libidinal cathexis on his father (who, in the film, is never mentioned), nor even on his childhood friend Buck, but his memories of the collaborative and erotic pleasures represented by the inventive dramas the two boys wrote and performed. As opposed to the plays he wrote and games he devised with Buck, which brought a sense of erotic and creative possibility, Chuck's current life is a round of anxiously maintained conventions, from the competitive bravado of his business deals, about which he cares too much, to the odd sterility of his emotional life, about which he seems to care too little. Heterosexuality, in the film, relies on the disavowed repression of creative sociality, producing in Chuck an emotional vacuity and unregulated ambition that keep him from forming meaningful social relationships, even "straight" ones, in the present. Carlyn admits to Buck that Chuck is "not very sentimental," adding, "He cares a lot about his work." Shutting out the sentiments associated with memory, Chuck is locked in a grim present, where he cares less about other people than he does about financial success, which he also seems to pursue without pleasure. Disavowing both his past and his grief over that past, the unsentimental Chuck is a painful example of the consequences of Butler's double repression, made ironic when we learn that his current work involves pursuing a band called Freudian.

Other models of psychosubjectivity at work in *Chuck & Buck,* however, involve substantially less unremembering. While the repressive Chuck is a Freudian, Buck, emphasizing the creative and erotic exuberance of childhood, is a Jungian. Setting himself up at the Aeternus Theater, across the street from Chuck's workplace, Buck is a "puer aeternus," the Jungian "eternal boy" who embodies narcissistic immaturity and a marked preference for fantasy over reality, but who is also capable of passionate attachments ("I'm waiting for my friend," Buck tells curious passersby as he stands outside the theater day after day staring at Chuck's office). While pursuing Chuck in Los Angeles, Buck lives in the Little Prince Motel, invoking what Marie-Louise von Franz, in her book *Puer Aeternus,* calls the ur-text of the puer aeternus tradition, Antoine de Saint-Exupery's classic anti-adulthood tale of childhood wisdom.[14]

As Saint-Exupery's *The Little Prince* attests, childhood has its powers, and so it proves in the film, in which Buck's dreamy, narcissistic pleasure principle proves less a drive than an overdrive, most subversive when seemingly most vulnerably innocent. In one potent example, Buck, appearing unannounced at Chuck's workplace, observes, "It's weird you have this office. What do you do in here?" to which Chuck defensively answers, "Sign bands and produce and negotiate contracts. It's not all that interesting." Buck's response insists on bringing memory into the place from which it has been banished. "That's really funny," Buck replies, "'cause you remember? We used to play games like we were businessmen. Remember we bought all those office supplies?" As Buck reminds him of their childhood games, Chuck nods as if he *is* starting to remember, and when Buck reaches his punch line — "Is it real now or is it still a game?" — the ambivalence of Chuck's response, "It's pretty real," situates him at the juncture between fantasy and reality that is Buck's habitual terrain. When Chuck's assistant interrupts to announce a call, his response, "I'll return," signals both the suspension of business-as-usual and the temporal elision triggered by Buck's insistence on remembering. The disruptive crises occasioned by Buck's memories become even more dangerous when they become explicitly eroticized. Showing up late one night at Carlyn and Chuck's home, Buck suggests that he and Chuck play a game. When Chuck asks, "What do you mean? Like Trivial Pursuit or something?" Buck replies, "Like one of those games where you stick your dick in my mouth and I stick mine in yours. Chuck and Buck. Suck and fuck."

However playfully inventive, memory, for Buck, is no game, no trivial pursuit. Rather, it is unpredictably insistent, captivatingly pleasurable, disruptively erotic, a disruptive intervention, in short, in the normativity that Chuck's unremembering seeks to safeguard.

While the exemplar of mature heterosexual masculinity may wish to chuck his past, he is, at best, able only to temporarily buck it, for its pleasures persist less in the external form of a childhood friend than in subjectivity-shaping (and unshaping and reshaping) pleasures that cannot be eliminated to purchase individual "normalcy" any more than they can be to achieve cultural "health." While Buck may seem the odd character in the film, the oddest behavior is, from start to finish, Chuck's. From his initial decision to attend Mrs. O'Brien's funeral, Chuck seems drawn to the past he insists he wants to forget, making Buck an occasion rather than an agent of his remembrance. Chuck seems to experience relief each time Buck forces him to acknowledge that "maturity" is not something one achieves once and for all but a tiresome labor of repeated repression that achieves only an apparent result. When, in response to Chuck's prescriptive, "You've got to grow up," Buck responds, "Like you?" Chuck's softened "I'm trying, you know" makes an appeal to connective sympathy. And when Chuck, exasperated by Buck's unannounced visits, tells Buck, "I know we were really good friends. Once. . . . But that was a long time ago. My life is really complicated right now. I've got a ton of work and I'm getting married," adding, "I can't deal with you. I'm not the same person anymore," he seems close to recognizing the labor ("I can't deal with you") that goes into the repressions necessary to make a "really complicated" life seem worth the effort. Although he tells Buck, "I don't know why you're fixated on me," the real question of the film is why Chuck—who for no clear reason agrees to go to Mrs. O'Brien's funeral, to spend a night in a hotel room with Buck, to have sex with Buck despite his claims to be a "different person," and then, after Buck agrees to leave him alone forever, to invite his old friend to his wedding—remains so fixated on Buck and all he represents.

While Chuck may be a soft sell on the merits of returning to the past, a therapeutic culture scaffolds and ensures his continual labor, assuring him that forgetting is the price of normative standards of maturity and health. In one of the few conversations he has with Carlyn, Buck, responding to her question about his childhood with Chuck, says, "When

we were kids we did those things . . . sex things." Carlyn's calm reply—
"I know all about that. Kids are kids. They experiment. It's completely
normal"—renders the past both distant and safe, a "stage" in childhood
development toward adult heterosexuality. Buck's response—"What happened wasn't normal"—is not a confession of shame but a refusal of Carlyn's
naturalizing imposition of a developmental paradigm onto his insistence
that the past is still *present* in his relationship with Chuck, who may be
less "normal" than Carlyn supposes. Ignoring this statement, she becomes more insistently therapeutic, claiming, "You know, Buck, I'm wor-
ried about you. You've lost your mother—that's *hard.*" Once again, Buck
refuses the hint at a psychoanalytic account of homosexuality, locating
his eroticism not in the absence of an overly cathected mother but in
the loss of a friend: "He started it," Buck insists. "He made me this way."
Carlyn's last resort reveals the temporal distance that has been her object
all along, as she tells Buck, "It was a long time ago," to which his childish response—"So?"—denies the *pastness* that suggests memory's irrele-
vance in the present. Carlyn, growing impatient, shifts to developmental
imperatives, telling Buck, "You need to let go. You have to create something new." For her, nostalgia is a pathological "holding on" and maturity
a clean break into "something new," a value-laden opposition Buck re-
sists, demonstrating a previously unrevealed analytic acumen: "You want
to act like I'm crazy. But the truth is, I was here way before you and I
know what you are. You're like his house and his car. That's all. Chuck
and me—he's all I have." Heterosexual maturity, in Buck's account, is not
"something new" but so conventional as to be one more commodity in a
catalog of normative fetishes. Of course, Carlyn's construction of developmental "newness" is paradoxical (how would the subject who creates
the "new" exist without memory from previous developmental stages?),
producing a crisis in normativity that Buck, with deft ingenuity, aggra-
vates by his insistence on remembering.

The power of memory comes from neither its pastness nor its recov-
erability but from its temporally uncertain and incomplete narratives.
These make memory a potentially collaborative and creative occasion for
forging alternative *presents* from crises in the naturalized and seemingly
inevitable chronologies of "normal" life. In *Chuck & Buck,* we do not
learn what "really" happened between the two boys through recuperative
memory (in the form, say, of filmic flashback) but through a multiply

fictional metanarrative: the play *Hank & Frank* that Buck writes to bring memory into the present as a performance rather than as mimetic recovery. With its barely discernible plot and incoherent tags of dialogue, the play's performance is a disjointed hodgepodge of collaborative imaginings, creation and interpretation, none of which relies on a retrievable past. But those experiences are themselves based in imaginative and collaborative fantasy (as Buck tells Chuck, he wrote the play "thinking about the plays we used to put on," implying that memory narratives take us not to a "real" past but to another moment of narrative). Adding additional layers of fantasy onto his memory-play, Buck models his script on the production currently being staged by the Aeternus Theater's child actors: Frank Baum's *The Wizard of Oz*. Baum's tale is an appropriate model, both because its over-the-top production values (Buck's play takes place in front of a stylish backdrop of the Emerald City, quoted from the movie) remind us that camp has traditionally recuperated the "trash" that the rest of the culture devalues (as it devalues the "simple" Buck) and because of the association of *The Wizard of Oz* with gay culture. As we argued in our second chapter, *The Wizard of Oz* depicts the restless investments in and escapes from homes and homelands: in Kansas Dorothy can dream only of Oz, but in Oz she wants to "go home" where, at the film's end, she imagines her Midwestern compatriots as the fantastical inhabitants of Oz. What spatial homelessness is for Dorothy, temporal displacement is for Buck, allowing neither past nor present to be a self-sufficient "home" but insisting that, however fictional and provisionary, both are necessary to the generation of collaborative community that releases one from the isolating solitude of "normalcy." If Dorothy is a character, like Buck, constantly in motion, she is also, like Buck, a purposeful dreamer who generates elaborate hybrids of reality and fantasy that make room for desires that those living, like Chuck, in the "real" world either repress or discredit.

At its conclusion, with the poisoned Frank and Hank dead in each other's arms like little queer Romeo and Juliets, Buck's play apparently leads to the tragic loss that would seem to be the inevitable trajectory of his quixotic attempt to rescue Chuck from his own unremembering. As with Gonzalez-Torres's *acedic* aesthetics, however, Buck's art is about idealism, not tragedy. The idealism embedded in the narrative of loss becomes clear in Buck's other artwork, which he produces for Chuck when

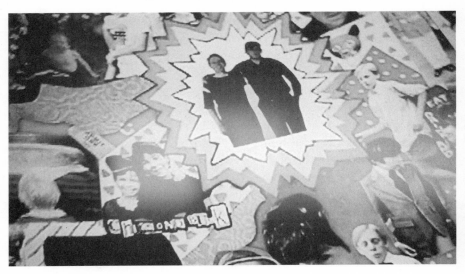

Collage from the film *Chuck & Buck,* 2000.

he discovers his friend has no photographs of them in his house. This collage, done in a style reminiscent of the 1970s, centers on a photograph of the two adult men with their arms around each other's shoulders, Chuck looking decidedly awkward. That central image is surrounded by photos of the boys as children framed by phrases like "summer fun" and "eat, drink, and be merry," all set on an explosion of bright colors and a collage of fabrics and patterns. Chuck's awkward discomfort (the photograph was taken, pointedly, in Chuck's business office) contrasts sharply with the exuberant pleasure evident in his childhood photos. Buck's artwork is an homage not only to his individual past but to a cultural past as well. The work resembles the photomontages of Gilbert and George, who similarly set photographs of men — often in sexualized positions — into fantastically colored environments. The resemblance between these aesthetics connects the seemingly naïve Buck to a gay erotic aesthetic. The photos of Chuck and Buck as children no longer signify, as Buck earlier says, that Chuck "is all I have" but reflect his ability to turn their relationship into a remembered aesthetic (an aesthetics *of* remembrance) that reflects that earlier friendship in other similar relationships (Chuck and Buck as Gilbert and George?) in the past and, presumably, in the future.

While in the center photo Chuck stares directly out at the viewer, Buck's photo stares not at Chuck, as we might expect, but in the opposite direction, outside the frame of the collage. His adult desires no longer need his childhood friend, his outward gaze suggests, having replaced a person who can bring only loss with an ideal that will persist beyond that loss.

Realizing the ideal of his photo collage, Buck's play *Hank & Frank* inadvertently generates the ideal community he has been yearning for all along. Written and produced for the sole purpose of telling Chuck something about their shared past, *Hank & Frank* — in which one boy seduces the other into "playing games" (presumably sexual) in the woods, leading to both boys being poisoned by an evil witch — is, on the most immediate level, a flop. True, Chuck does seem to recognize his counterpart who says, "You keep talking about that night, but I just don't remember," only to end by confessing his love for his dying friend. One could speculate that Chuck's ultimate decision to accompany Buck to his hotel room and then have sex with his childhood love is the result of his interpellation into Buck's staged fantasy. Ultimately, however, although plays and art cannot recuperate the past, they can do something even better: they can carry an ideal, cloaked in loss, from the past in order to generate a more pleasurable present.

That is, indeed, what happens to Buck. Even while grieving the loss of his hopes for recapturing Chuck's love, Buck comes to recognize that what that relationship meant to him — creativity, erotic play, companionship, solace — are still available in more bountiful forms. Buck does get his nominal object of desire when, asking Chuck, "Do you remember me?" his old friend responds, "Yeah, I remember you. I remember everything." In the meantime, though, Buck has learned to dream bigger dreams. Despite much sadness (he four times breaks down in tears during the film), Buck learns that memory is not a way back to the past but the means to establish alternatives in a present shared with an expandable and imaginative community willing to open themselves emotionally despite differences of identity, aesthetics, and values. The new friends Buck makes while producing *Hank & Frank* share a compassionate acceptance that comes from their alienation from the normalcy exhaustingly maintained by Chuck and Carlyn. One of the actors, the down-and-out Sam, praises Buck for writing "a fantastic play" and invites him to move into an apartment across the hall, while the office-manager-turned-director, Beverly, provides the recognition Chuck withholds. Early on, in response to his habitual question, "Do you remember me?" Beverly pleases Buck by responding, "It's the man who's waiting for his friend." Later, heartbroken by Chuck, Buck, crying on Beverly's shoulder, says, "There's no love for me. Not anymore," but she assures him, "Yes there is."

The hopeful idealism that can promise future love comes not from denying memory but from transforming memories into an ideally compassionate subculture. Sam and Beverly are able to provide encouragement and consolation because they are as perverse and quirky as Buck. Sam, when he first visits Buck's motel room, initially seems put off by the childhood décor, declaring, "It's like fucking Romper Room in here. There's something funny about you. You funny?" Rather than erupting into homophobic violence, however, Sam quickly adds, "I'm funny too." Later, when Buck confesses to Beverly, "I'm afraid of a lot of things, you know," she replies, "I am too. . . . Lots of things. I'm a *mess.*" The bonds that come from being "funny" or a "mess" — of living life with the memory of alienation from "real life" — allow Buck to move beyond trying to recapture the imaginative collaborations of his childhood. The film ends with the suggestion that Buck can start to turn the memories of those emotions into new kinds of bonds. In the film's last scene at Chuck and Carlyn's wedding reception, a gay-coded man says to Buck, "I like wedding cake," to which Buck replies, "Me too. It's sweet." Buck's response, at once erotically suggestive and childishly innocent, suggests that his characteristic conflations of sex and simplicity have found their milieu and that, now the object rather than the subject of desire, he may be on the verge of new adventures. Without denying the traumatic loss represented by Chuck's marriage, Buck manages to retain his ideals not in the past but in the present, not in a single object but in a varied and collaborative community, and not in memory but *through* memory into the present. Feeling backward but moving forward, Buck manages to have his cake and eat it, too.

Although *Chuck & Buck* makes no explicit reference to the gay cultural past, much less to AIDS, both might well be understood in relationship to the film's investigation of loss and idealism and how memory can hold communities together even in the face of crisis. Divided between a past characterized by campy whimsy and sexual adventure and a present characterized by an anxious normalcy purchased through willed forgetting, *Chuck & Buck* seems structured by the dynamics of de-generational unremembering that plagued gay culture in the years preceding the film's release.[15] The traumatic break between Chuck and Buck echoes the divide in gay culture between the pre-AIDS decade characterized, like Buck, as unsophisticated, nostalgic, immature, narcissistic, whimsical, misogynistic, aggressive, unrealistic, and highly stylized, and the post-AIDS decades characterized, like Chuck, in terms of a willed and anxious commitment to normalcy at the expense of memory. Whereas conventional narratives of this historical rupture insist that gay men need to choose, once and for all, between pleasure or normalcy, memory or health, Buck refuses to choose, making memory the ampersand that keeps his recollection and idealism, one impossible without the other, in continual proximity. Bringing innocence and innovation, sexual desire and friendships, across seemingly unbridgeable historical divides, Buck provides a model for how people living in the continuing devastation of AIDS can resist both mainstream imperatives to forget and queer claims that memory can lead only to shame, abjection, and antisocial isolation, choosing instead the ideals necessary to community formation and collective change persistently at the heart of ideality politics.

Remains to Be Seen

When Buck learns to use memory to engage others in an idealistic imagination in the present and for the future, he enacts what filmmaker Alexandra Juhasz calls "queer archival activism." Juhasz's poignant and powerful *Video Remains* (2005) enacts this strategy by combining footage of the filmmaker's college friend Jim Lamb, who died from AIDS in 1993; videotaped interviews with members of the Los Angeles queer youths of color group Mpowerment; and voice-overs drawn from telephone conversations between Juhasz and various female friends about memory and filmmaking, mortality and activism. The video burns with the imperative to remember and the frustrating inadequacy of efforts to do so. "I can't say I'm honoring peoples' memories well enough," Juhasz says in the voice-over, acknowledging, "One always fails in the face of that responsibility." Yet, as Juhasz also shows, her "failure" becomes a temporal disjuncture between experience and memory, past and present, that allows for imaginative shaping and even correction on the part of survivors. The "failure" of memory, in short, enables the success of filmmaking, of *vision* in both senses, in ways that fuse idealism with loss and make them explicit as articulate aspirations for action on behalf of a more just and fulfilling future.

Juhasz's project begins from the problem of unremembering that has concerned us in this book: that by the end of the 1990s, people were unremembering AIDS and the communities lost to AIDS, and with that unremembering came the end of activism and of communities held together by forms of activism enabled by memory. As Juhasz's friend Alisa Lebov laments, "One of the things that seems to be true, I don't know about the '90s but certainly the 2000s, is that we've almost stopped talking about it [AIDS] with one another, and that's how you and I met, that's how I *know* you." The video begins as a way to fill that gap. Novelist Sarah Schulman (whose *People in Trouble* is another powerful example of idealist memory) assures Juhasz, "When these people are dead, and when I am dead, these interviews will still exist, and people will be able to go back and see that . . . there was an active gay movement and an active gay community that supported people with AIDS who were abandoned by straight people and their families and their government. And that was the true dynamic, though it hasn't yet been shown." Despite this promise, the capacity of contemporary viewers to "go back" is challenged by the fact that, as another friend puts it, "the video is so alive and the people are so dead."

But even when we do remember, the project of memory is frustrated by the sometimes startling divergence between our recollections of people or events and the way they are captured on film. Although one of Juhasz's friends wants to find in her memories of those who have died "all this wisdom" and "amazing poetry," Juhasz's friend Jim, whom she describes as "a crazy, lying, wild, brilliant, dynamic man" who "died in a state of unfulfilled chaos, which is how he lived," refuses the dignified profundity that memory often craves. Although Jim "wanted to be recorded speaking great insight and poetry," his incoherent and often self-involved narratives strike Juhasz as "very tragic," leading her — and the viewer — to feel ambivalence toward "these video tapes that stand in for memories." In *Video Remains,* the past is neither poetic nor profound, nor is memory complete or ever-present.

Idealism relies on neither poetry nor profundity, however, and the incompleteness of memory becomes an occasion for inventive collaboration on the part of those who remember. Because of this, *Video Remains* is strikingly, if critically, optimistic. A story told by hairstylist Michael Anthony sums up what "remains" after friends have passed. When he offered to vacuum the "dust bunnies" left in the apartment after his vocal coach, a transvestite named Alexandra, packed to move to a hospital where she would die from AIDS, Alexandra tells him, "Leave them there for all the memories of all the good times we had here. Throw them in the air so the next person will remember what it was like when we had our great get-togethers and our parties and our great moments of intimate conversation and planning for other things in our lives and our goals." Memories, translated into the most mundane form of "remains" — dust — persist as a continual reminder to Anthony — as to the others interviewed in the video — of his love for people in the past. Above all, it reminds them that "we stuck by them," that a collective ethos once existed, contrary to the present characterizations of the past as self-involved and uncaring.

Juhasz articulates that collective ethos in an essay occasioned by *Video Remains* in which she describes the inventive memory-transforming work of what she calls nostalgia. Rejecting the conventional conceptions of nostalgia as a "paltry and passive" sentiment and acknowledging that "dreaming a past that is always better, never attainable, and by no means true" can be "wretched and pitiable," Juhasz nevertheless contends that nostalgia can be "a yearning shared by a community of others" and hence a potent incentive for activism ("Video Remains," 321–23). "One generation's yearning could fuel another's learning," she writes, "if we could look back together and foster an escape from melancholia through productive, communal nostalgia" (323). Video, Juhasz argues, is a particularly valuable antidote to melancholia, which she dismisses as pathologizing and paralyzing, because it preserves the past. At the same time, Juhasz acknowledges her role as a video artist in shaping archival materials, transforming pastness, through a "sensuous engagement with the material" (323), into something better suited to the needs of the present, "a more adaptive, contextual, and living kind of lasting" (326). Essential to this collectivizing function is the infusion into archival materials of "feelings of desire, love, hope, or despair" (326), the intangible emotions that, as we stated at the outset, conventional histories neglect but which are central to what Gregg Bordowitz calls the "affective condition of political activism."[16] Keenly aware that "good politics of representation" are not enough to "forestall the bad political-economic-material conditions of biology, presidential disavowal, and the capitalist imperatives of the pharmaceutical industry" (325), Juhasz nevertheless maintains her faith in visual arts that enable us "to remember, feel anew, analyze, and educate, ungluing the past from its melancholic grip, and instead living it as a gift with others in the here and now" (326).

To turn a vision into that collectivizing pedagogy requires its representation as loss, which asserts that having once existed ("so you can prove that it was there," as Juhasz says), ideals are attainable and may once again exist. But our desire for what has been lost must not lead us to misunderstand the constitutive relationship of memory and idealism but rather to conceive the forward-looking idealism behind memory (as Juhasz observes, "The nostalgic romance is not with a fantasy" but, rather, with an idealism based on real and attainable longings [323]). Fantasy, especially the social fantasy we are calling idealism, is what transforms "a mournful love for the past" into "a public, hopeful, future-looking project" (324) that "looks not just to an indexical trace of the past but creates the possibility for an anticipated trace of the future" (326). That idealism can take the form, in Juhasz's words, of "living our lives as responsibly and responsively as we can, and continuing activism on any level, on any issue, is to me a way that we can honor those lives." To do that requires the creativity of filmmakers like Juhasz, the collaboration of her friends like Anthony, Shulman, and Lebov, and the objects of memory, however incomplete or flawed, like Jim. But above all it requires an idealism realistic about the materiality of loss and the persistence of ambivalence, yet persistent, adaptive, and hopeful. Especially as queer theory moves beyond the collectivizing—but sometimes essentializing and homogenizing—power of identity, memory's ideality politics stand out as a crucial tool to counter the hold of normative inevitability and, reckoning with the past, to engage creatively in collective activism on behalf of "accountability and justice" for ourselves in the present and for the future. With Felix Gonzalez-Torres, Mike White, and Alex Juhasz, we claim for memory neither transparent detachment nor affective accuracy, but rather aspiration cloaked in the narrative conventions of recollection and loss. Only when critical detachment joins with affect and desire to create ideal imaginings can the full work of progressive remembering be carried forth by and for those for whom the values associated with that past promise a more just and pleasurable present and for whom the very *pastness* of those values, the claim that they once existed, legitimize the optimistic faith that they might exist again. If memory serves, they will.

ACKNOWLEDGMENTS

"Memory," Oscar Wilde wrote, "is the diary that chronicles things that never happened or couldn't possibly have happened." Throughout this book we endorse Wilde's sense of the extravagant fancy often associated with memories, but we are also fortunate to have memories of very real acts of kindness and generosity. For discussing ideas with us, reading drafts, making valuable recommendations, and inviting us to try out portions of the book while still in progress, we remember with real gratitude Martin Berger, David Bergman, Michael Camille, Russ Castronovo, George Chauncey, Tina Chen, Charlotte Eubanks, Susan Gillman, Leigh Gilmore, Ron Gregg, Barbara Greene and her colleagues at Notre Dame, Larry Gross and his colleagues at Penn, David Halperin, Sharon Haar, Eric Hayot, Andrew Hostetler, Alex Juhasz, Jonathan Katz, Jongwoo Kim, Christopher Lane, Jeff Masten, Richard Morrison, Anthony Musillami, Dana Nelson, Eden Osucha and her colleagues at Bates, Don Pease, Beth Povinelli, Eric Rofes, Alan Sinfield, Marc Stein, and Jonathan Walz. We are especially grateful to Beth Freeman, Dana Luciano, and a third anonymous reader who provided us with invaluable detailed and constructive commentary on the entire manuscript. A fellowship from the Gay and Lesbian Alliance Against Defamation Center for the Study of Media and Society enabled our research on *Will and Grace.* We are grateful to GLAAD, especially to center director Van Cagle for his guidance and support.

We are deeply thankful to Robin Schulze, head of the English department, and Susan Welch, dean of the College for the Liberal Arts, both of whom have supported our scholarship and made Penn State a delightful place to be working scholars. For his never-ending affection, his dizzying erudition, and his own particular form of queer optimism, we thank Robert Caserio. From the start of this project, we received the richest and most thoughtful feedback from Richard Morrison, first as an extraordinarily astute reader, then as a valued friend, and finally as the best guide we could hope for in the completion of this project. We threatened Richard that we would thank him for being much funnier than you would expect an editor to be; for that, and much, much more, we are grateful to him and also to the staff at the University of Minnesota Press.

Finally, to the three men to whom the book is dedicated — brilliant, brave gay men and generous, gentle mentors — we owe our sense of the possible, as do all people who read and empathize with this book.

NOTES

Introduction

1. "My Guide to Queer Memphis," http://www.angelfire.com/tn/queermemphis/insiders.html.

2. Alasdair MacIntyre, *After Virtue,* 221, as quoted and discussed in Younge, "White History 101," 10.

3. This book makes no claims to speak for or about lesbian identities conceived as distinct from sexual identities that include men, although this disclaimer should not be interpreted to suggest either that lesbians have produced no memory narratives or that women are irrelevant to our interests. On the contrary, we have been deeply inspired by lesbian artists and theorists, many of whom are cited and discussed in the following chapters. We mean our focus on gay men, a group with which we have particular identifications and investments, to be a case study of the constituency singled out by de-generational unremembering in the aftermath of AIDS, not a claim for cultural exceptionality. Just as there have been distinct but mutually informing histories of gay and of lesbian culture, we hope that this study will complement, not foreclose, similar work on lesbian memory narratives.

4. See also Huyssen, *Present Pasts.* The "hypertrophy of memory" Huyssen claims to identify here brings with it its own form of forgetting, a "memory

fatigue" induced by "excess and saturation in the marketing of memory" (3; see also 17). Huyssen is concerned with two strands of "the current memory narrative": first, a broad context that includes "the mass-marketing of nostalgia" in the form of "retro fashions and repro furniture," "obsessive self-musealization per video recorder, memoir writing," historical fiction, and popular documentaries such as the programming on the History Channel (a lumping together of phenomena that might be more profitably investigated in their particularity) and second, what seems to be his real focus, "the ever more ubiquitous Holocaust discourse" (14), about which he has a great deal that is interesting and specific to say.

5. On the rhetoric of de-generational unremembering from the Christian right in the 1990s, see Burlein. Three of the "five bad ideas" Focus on the Family founder and president James Dobson attributed to the 1960s are associated with sex/gender norms: "the sexual revolution, feminism, [and] divorce." The other two are drugs and "'God is dead' theology" (Burlein, "Countermemory on the Right," 209).

6. For a cogent analysis of these crackdowns and their consequences for queer sexual culture, see Berlant and Warner, "Sex in Public," and Warner, *The Trouble with Normal*.

7. Muñoz's defensiveness concerning his engagement with the era of the sexual revolution contrasts with his willingness to confront other shibboleths of established queer theory, specifically its "romance of singularity and negativity" (10), with which his ideals of collective utopia are refreshingly at odds.

8. See Edelman, *No Future*. Defending generational models, Elizabeth Freeman writes, "Though some feminists have advocated abandoning the generational model because it relies on family as its dominant metaphor and identity as the commodity it passes on, the concept of generations linked by political work or even by mass entertainment also acknowledges the ability of various culture industries to produce shared subjectivities that go beyond the family" ("Packing History, Count(er)ing Generations," 729).

9. Tim Dean's study of barebacking culture, *Unlimited Intimacy*, opens by insisting that this practice does not recall pre-AIDS sexuality: "Unprotected anal sex between men has become something different than it once was: barebacking does not represent a 'relapse' or a misguided return to what gay sex before AIDS used to be" (5). Though this rejection of the recent past is reiterated — "Fifteen years ago, a statement that explicitly characterized unsafe sex as a viable option would have been unthinkable.... Now, however, this announcement figures unprotected sex as a deliberate choice for which the individual must take responsibility" (117) — it is not analyzed. Dean's analysis makes clear that barebackers

are not forgetting AIDS; the virus is central to the ethos of "bug chasers" and the kinship networks of infection Dean argues characterize barebacking culture. Rather, what is being aggressively unremembered is the ethos "of protection and thus of mutual care" (5) that characterized gay sex culture's response to AIDS in the 1980s and early 1990s. Dean does not address barebackers' attitudes toward that sex culture, preferring to contrast their opinions with what he calls the "conservative" attitudes of other gay men, which he characterizes in terms of their advocacy of gay marriage. Nor does Dean address how barebacking culture emerged historically in relation to ideologies of safer sex. The absence of history from this account is a consequence of Dean's problematic insistence that readers suspend moral judgment about barebacking by treating it as a "homology" (30) with psychoanalysis (that is, a field of psychic drives and patterns that elicit "psychoanalytic neutrality" [28] rather than judgment) and as a "foreign culture" that deserves an anthropological form of "care and respect" (x) from observers seeking to understand its folkways: "Like any culture, this one has its own language, rituals, etiquette, institutions, iconography, and so on" (x). These models, as deployed by Dean, elide consideration of memory: psychoanalytic drives are construed as timeless, and his list of issues anthropologists engage conspicuously avoids origin myths or the role of ancestors. Barebackers' attitudes toward the safe-sex advocates of "fifteen years ago" just go unconsidered. Are they contemptuous? Angry? Dismissive? Or—and this is the implication of Dean's silence on the topic—has safe-sex culture simply been unremembered. Thus, Dean's study— brilliant as it frequently is—exemplifies the propensity for unremembering in contemporary queer theory.

10. Notable exceptions, to which we are very indebted, are Douglas Crimp's *Melancholia and Moralism* and Ann Cvetkovich's *An Archive of Feelings*, both of which are powerful analyses of the trauma of AIDS and the kinds of remembering and memorialization that are possible in its wake.

11. Israel Rosenfeld's *The Invention of Memory* summarizes the evidence that memory is a dynamic process of categorization of experience and conjecture dependent on "individual needs and desires" (166). Marita Sturken's "Narratives of Recovery" offers an overview of debates around repressed/recovered memory syndrome attentive to the ways that American culture has fetishized personal memory in an era of "cultural forgetting" (243), raising the possibility that individual abuse memories (whether "true" or not) stand in as, in Carol Tavris's words, a "'brilliant figurative metaphor' for the powerlessness that women feel" (240). For an overview of more recent "hindsight research," which documents people's tendency to remember predicting what they now know to have happened, see Baruch Fischhoff, "An Early History of Hindsight Research."

12. John D'Emilio establishes the connections between industrial capitalism and gay identity, writing, "In divesting the household of its economic independence and fostering the separation of sexuality from procreation, capitalism has created conditions that allow some men and women to organize a personal life around their erotic/emotional attraction to their own sex" ("Capitalism and Gay Identity," 7).

13. For a fuller discussion of how reformable traits became associated with homosexuality in this period, see Castiglia, *Interior States*.

14. On the consolidation of the "dandy" into the "homosexual," see Reed, *Art and Homosexuality*, 95–97.

15. Among theorists working in fields related to this project, an interesting division of labor appears. Critics addressing race tend to focus on questions related to memory, in which the problem becomes an overinscription of memory by official historiographic sources that impose linear progression onto divergent events so as to piece together an account of increased freedom more pleasing to those in power than fair to the recollections and experiences of those whose history is purportedly told. This is true of the work of Nyong'o, Muñoz, and E. Patrick Johnson, who poignantly figures (and refigures) the remembered past as "home" in ways reminiscent of other African American writers. Critics writing on lesbianism (mostly distinct from questions of race), on the other hand, have focused largely on temporality and its reversals, ruptures, and remappings rather than on memory per se. This work tends to share with broader theorizations of time and memory a sense of the problematic linearity of progressive time, although disruptions of time in these works have less to do with divergent recollections than with sexual experience (as in Elizabeth Freeman's remarkable account of S/M's queer time), with a notion of "queer time" abstracted from human agency and socially embedded practices, or with textual expression in the past (as in Heather Love's incisive account of "bad feelings" in late-nineteenth- and early-twentieth-century American literature). Heather Love's *Feeling Backward* is particularly interesting in this regard. Focusing on the negative affects that haunt queer sexuality, feelings such as shame, loss, sadness, Love provides a valuable corrective to the often overidealizing positivity of much liberation writing and its subsequent rendering in history. Love is right to remind us that the past can be a downer, but that that, too, can enable the kinds of activism in the present that we attribute to memory. Against these critical developments, we focus on memory rather than abstract time as a site of historically specific discursive contentions and attend to sources other than the literary and to affects other than the negative. We also see "memory" as a more constructed than transparent relation to the past and examine the effects of *pastness* theoretically.

16. See, for instance, "Friendship as a Way of Life."

17. Muñoz is similarly critical of Bersani's influential "anti-social queer theories," which foreclose the "utopian hopes and possibilities" he is interested in (*Cruising Utopia*, 11, 34).

1. Battles over the Gay Past

1. See, for example, Crain, "Pleasure Principles"; Stolberg, "Gay Culture Weighs Sense and Sexuality"; Vaid, "Last Word"; and Warner, "Media Gays."

2. Rotello and Signorile were columnists for *New York Newsday* and the *New York Times*, respectively, while Sullivan was editor of the *New Republic* from 1991 to 1996, before being hired as a writer for the *New York Times Magazine*. Other neoconservative columnists of the era include Eddie James, winner of the 1997–98 Randy Shilts Award for Outstanding Achievement, who began his column for the *Baltimore Alternative* (February 1998), "Sex & Sensibility: Why Are Some Men Losing the Latex?" with this frankly de-generational linkage of memory and unsafe sex: "John Travolta, Boogie Nights, disco balls, bell-bottoms — everywhere you look the signs are painfully clear that the '70s are back. And among gay men, a small but growing number are not just embracing the pop cultural kitsch of the polyester era, they are also adopting its pre-AIDS, anything-goes mentality when it comes to sex."

3. Michael Warner has argued that gay neoconservatives "repudiate the legacies of the gay movement — its democratic conception of activism, its goal of political mobilization, its resistance to the regulation of sex and its aspiration to a queer world." This repudiation of the 1970s' legacy allows gay neocons to "promote a vision of the gay future as assimilation, and they willingly endorse state regulation of sex to that end. They are interested in sex only insofar as it lends itself to respectability and self-esteem; and forget unconscious desire, or the tension between pleasure and normalization, or the diversity of contacts through which queers have made a world for one another" ("Media Gays" 15).

4. Why gay men would want to serve the interests of a "general public" that has made little effort to serve gay interests is a complex question, and not one we can fully answer. On the most banal level, gay men, as AIDS activists and theorists have long pointed out, are part of that "general public," which not only entitles us (theoretically) to civil rights and police protection but frequently makes us agents as well as objects of mainstream thought. De-generation is also partially understandable in light of the fear that led many gay men in the early years of the epidemic, when safer sex education was scarce and changed rapidly, to conceive of celibacy or monogamy as the only viable responses to a sexually transmitted virus. One could argue as well that gay men, shocked at the decimation of a subculture they had worked so hard to create and by the deaths of those

with whom they inhabited it, have sought to defend themselves by minimalizing the value of what was lost. Finally, there is an implied prophylactic syllogism of blame: if the sexual revolution caused illness, and one distances oneself from the sexual revolution, one is therefore distanced from illness (Crimp, "Mourning and Militancy").

5. On attacks by the queer-identified group Sex Panic on Rotello and Signorile, see Crain, "Pleasure Principles." Rotello, like other gay journalists who advocate assimilation and invite government regulation, has been called a "turd" by Sex Panic and "neoconservative" by Michael Warner, who, in his July 1997 editorial "Media Gays" in *The Nation*, exhorts queers to ignore Rotello and to heed instead a host of queer theorists including Leo Bersani. Warner and Berlant cite "Is the Rectum a Grave?" in "Sex in Public," 566. On the queer aesthetics of *The Living End*, see Bronski, "Reel Politick."

6. As Michael Snediker pithily puts it, "One doesn't really shatter when one is fucked, despite Bersani's accounts of it" (*Queer Optimism*, 12).

7. Bersani presents his view of sex as justified both by biology ("anatomical considerations") and the universalized claims of Freudian psychology ("for the idea of penis envy describes how men feel about having one") (216). Bersani's denial that his is "an 'essentialist' view of sexuality" is premised on a definition of essentialism as "a priori, ideologically motivated, and prescriptive" (216). The ideologically motivated and prescriptive nature of his text we elucidate outside this note. His claims to have deduced the characteristics of sexuality a posteriori (as it were) rely on a central characteristic of essentialism: a false assertion of universalism that extrapolates the meaning(s) of sex from simplistic claims that "the reproduction of the species has most generally been accomplished by the man's getting on top of the woman," which implies a dynamic of "mastery and subordination" so totalizing that "for the woman to get on top is just a way of letting her play the game of power for awhile" so that "even on the bottom, the man can still concentrate his deceptively renounced aggressiveness in the thrusting movement of his penis," a proposition that is proved to Bersani's satisfaction by his experience with porn films (216).

8. Bersani's focus on anal intercourse and his metaphoric transformation of it into normative straight sex can be contextualized through Cindy Patton's description of how the 1986 "Heterosexual AIDS Panic" dramatically changed public discourse about safe sex: "Since among heterosexuals, or at least in the public culture of heterosexual men, penile-vaginal intercourse is the hegemonic and identity-creating act, the meaning of safe sex shifted toward abstinence, monogamy, and the use of condoms" (*Inventing AIDS*, 47). The heterosexualization of AIDS in the mainstream media then changed sexual discourse in the gay male community, where after 1986 "safe sex discussions inevitably began with a

discussion of the importance of condoms, and only then discussed the range of other possibilities for a fulfilling sex life" (48). While Patton's description of the heterosexualization of AIDS may help account for Bersani's sexual metaphors, it also renders more suspicious the alignment of gay male sexuality with "the public culture of heterosexual men." Similarly investigating Bersani's naturalization of anal sex as the missionary position, Michael Lucey wonders "whether by assuming the abject position the gender binary has constructed, the reactivation and perpetuation of that structure could be so definitively resisted—just as one might wonder if one particular way of having sex (and one particular way of imagining what is going on in that act) would be the most analytically evident route to such an end" (*Gide's Bent*, 89).

9. Michael Lucey astutely analyzes how Bersani's presentation of a "pure" sex act existing solely in the present is undermined ironically by the very acts—of remembering (inherent in writing) and of projecting a utopian moment when the rectum shatters the ego—that Bersani chastises in others: "When one writes about sex it is not so easy, no matter how hard one wriggles, to distinguish between past, future, and present, between reminiscences, anticipation, and enjoyment. One could write about sex for years and never get to a pure present without politics. Bersani's shattering present is ultimately inseparable from and even indistinguishable from the past and the future. It carries with it the structure of its own nostalgia" (40).

10. We are indebted to David Halperin for his insightful analysis of the possibilities for queer politics opened up by Foucault's writings on history; see his *Saint Foucault*, especially 104–6.

11. Willy's interaction with Alberto, the minor nonwhite character in the film, correctly described by Román as "unresolved," might be read as a painfully accurate encapsulation of the often mutually frustrating relationship among the different constituencies most affected by AIDS. What Román (following Watney) analyzes as the intemperate response of white critics who condemned the film for not living up to an ideal of inclusivity suggests how intensely this issue continued to rankle.

12. We share with Román the experience of "being incredibly moved" (290) by the conclusion of *Longtime Companion*, and being frustrated by the near-ubiquity of its critical vilification, which we attempted to counter in Castiglia, "Sex Panics," 170–71.

2. For Time Immemorial

1. "Between Memory and History" was an influential early translation of Nora's introductory text. Its appearance in the prestigious theory journal *Representations*

sanctioned for national identity a muddle of ideas that would have been subject to excoriating scrutiny had they been advanced in relation to sexual identity.

2. The *House Rules* exhibition catalog was published as *Assemblage* 24 (August 1994).

3. See, for instance, Chauncey, *Gay New York;* Newton, *Cherry Grove, Fire Island;* Stein, *City of Sisterly and Brotherly Loves.*

4. The two best accounts of this underexamined episode are James Saslow's funny and thoughtful "A Sculpture without a Country" and an account by one of the models, David B. Boyce.

5. On Peter Putnam, see entries for "Mildred Andrews Fund" and "Putnam, Mildred Olive Andrews and Peter Andrews Putnam," Encyclopedia of Cleveland History, http://ech.cwru.edu/ech-cgi.

6. The construction of the avant-garde in opposition to queer identities is treated at greater length in Reed, *Art and Homosexuality.*

7. Saslow preserved Nevelson's anonymity here but uses her name when he tells the same story in *Pictures and Passions,* 287.

8. This translation was offered by Karin Daan (personal correspondence, July 20, 2009).

9. Karin Daan, personal correspondence, July 20, 2009.

10. Each side of the granite triangles is ten meters long; each side of the triangular area marked out by the whole monument is thirty-six meters long. A 1987 informational flyer about the *Homomonument* expands the allusions to oppression beyond the historical specifics associated with the pink triangle, noting that, "Oppression of homosexuality existed long before the Nazis and continues to the present day."

11. Similar language was used in informational flyers about the project printed in 1987.

12. The *Homomonument*'s relationship to Jewish memory is complicated. The press conference announcing the winning design was held at the Anne Frank house, and Daan describes the author of the quotation inscribed in the marble, Jacob Israël de Haan, as "an Amsterdam Homosexual Jewish Poet" in the context of noting that the triangle with the text inscription "is pointing straight to the Anne Frank House" (personal correspondence, July 20, 2009). In the poem, "The Fisherman," however, de Haan attributes the "unmeasurable longing" for friendship to a handsome young fisherman encountered on a seaside holiday (Doyle). And de Haan occupies a fraught place in the history of Jewish letters, as his career spans both the scandalous homoeroticism of his early poetry—said to be the first explicitly homoerotic writing in Dutch—and his assassination in Palestine in 1924 by Zionists whose project of realizing a Jewish homeland he opposed (http://en.wikipedia.org/wiki/Jacob_Israël_de_Haan, citing Shlomo Nakdimon

and Shaul Mayzlish, *De Haan: ha-retsah ha-politi ha-rishon be-Erets Yisraël [De Haan: The first political assassination in Palestine]* [Tel Aviv: Modan Press, 1985]).

13. The flyer can be downloaded at http://www.homomonument.nl; for more information on the *Homomonument,* see also http://european-architecture.info/HOLLAND/AMS-S07. The symbolism associated with the present and future is multivalent. The commission jury described the raised triangle as "a podium . . . for those involved in the fight" and the stepped-down triangle pointing into the canal as "positioned to catch a favourable wind" (quoted in Koenders, *Het Homomonument,* 42), which might seem to correspond to the present and future respectively. Daan also describes the triangle pointing toward the political headquarters as a "podium": "It's a place to fight from and for! If necessary!" but she associates this with the future and describes the "watercornertriangle pointing straight to the Dam Square" as making "a connection to the Dam and the 'Dam Sleepers' in the Eighties, a sublime Amsterdam meeting-point" (personal correspondence).

14. On the populations and activities associated with the piers, see Sember, "In the Shadow of the Object," 230. Sember's thoughtful essay does not address the relationship of these visual markings to his themes of loss and remembrance. On Tava, see WWW.VINNYSNET presents TAVA'S PIER MURALS, http://www.vinnys.net/home/intrototheartist.html.

15. In a lecture delivered twice during the controversy over the Halsted Street markers, John Ricco defined queerness as manifest in "anonymous places" — "alleyways, parked cars, tearooms, bathhouse labyrinths, cruising grounds" — which are "unnameable, unformalizable, unrepresentable places outside of the law." He straightforwardly acknowledged that fleeting, anonymous sex may be no more conducive to "social cohesion and political expression" than it is to architecture ("The Itinerancy of Erotic Uncertainty"). See also Ricco, "Coming Together." For other examples of theorists celebrating these spaces, see Bell, "One-Handed Geographies"; Mark Robbins's installation "Scoring the Park," exhibited in *Disappeared,* curated by John Ricco at the Randolph Street Gallery, Chicago, 1996; and Urbach, "Spatial Rubbing." Far from being outside the law, public bathrooms in particular may be the most mapped, explicated, and policed of all spaces associated with sexual identity: Laud Humphrey's 1975 *Tearoom Trade* is a classic text in both the canon of sexology and sociological method (for the questions it raised about participant observation); for a more recent analysis of how the physical and social structures of men's rooms function to police homosexuality, see Edelman, "Men's Room."

16. For more on Holocaust memorials in Germany and derivatives of their visual vocabularies elsewhere, see Huyssen, *Present Pasts.*

17. Crout's complex project, partially and temporarily realized in 1993, is described in his "Wasting Architecture."

18. The presence of the naked and near-naked figures in the presentation photographs is not noted in the texts describing *Utopian Prospect*, which present the piece as being about the view from the structure (Robbins, *Angles of Incidence*, 9–10, 39).

19. What look like windows in the unexplicated illustration of Crout's model published by Betsky (186) are intended as "grossly exaggerated weep holes" that are meant to be filled with memorials dedicated to particular people, which is an interesting idea, but these shrines-in-weep-holes are then perceived through "a peephole" (Crout, "Wasting Architecture," 16, 19).

20. Jencks first invoked "what is locally called the gay eclectic style" to describe "the work of another interior decorator gone exterior" in "Fetishism in Architecture," *Architectural Design*, August 1976, 493. Quotations are from his influential *The Language of Post-Modern Architecture*, 66; and *Daydream Houses of Los Angeles*, 11–12. "Gay eclectic" also appears in his "Genealogy of Post-Modern Architecture," 271. For a more appreciative and detailed analysis of this architecture, see Chase, *Exterior Decoration*.

21. Insistence on the invisibility of queer space guaranteed itself by proscribing acknowledgment that the queerness of design could be recognized. In Ronald Kraft's 1993 profile of openly gay Los Angeles architect Brian Murphy, known for his Astroturf-covered kitchen counters and chandeliers made from policemen's flashlights among other extravagant whimsies, Betsky is quoted warning Kraft off an interpretation of these as an expression of sexual identity: "If one were to find a gay sensibility in Murphy, it would only confirm the worst clichés of gay design — that they take serious art and turn it into eye candy. It is the cliché of the gay man as promiscuous not only sexually but also visually." It was left to one of the architect's straight clients to celebrate the idea that "the most outrageous drag queen would feel completely comfortable in the house Brian built for us" ("This Gay House," 58).

22. This instance is quoted from Peake ("Race and Sexuality," 426), where it is contrasted with the "high visibility" of commercial spaces in "many gay male ghettos." Although Peake's description of a lesbian enclave in Grand Rapids, Michigan, describes street parties, a restaurant, plans for more businesses, and an organizer's concern to "keep the streetscape intact" (427), none of this registers as visibility. This blinkered analysis is raised to a point of principle by Gill Valentine, whose study of a lesbian neighborhood that she keeps anonymous (itself an imposition of invisibility) asserts that "like Peake's study of lesbian neighborhoods in Grand Rapids . . . there are no lesbian businesses, retail outlets or bars in the neighborhood . . . like the lesbian neighborhood in Grand Rapids, [it] is an invisible ghetto. There are no public expressions of lesbian sexualities; no mark on the landscape that 'lesbians live here'" ("Out and About," 99). A near-identical

passage reappears in Valentine's coauthored introduction to Bell and Valentine's *Mapping Desire* (6). By claiming invisibility as the paradigm for lesbian community, however, Valentine avoids analyzing norms she seems to have internalized in her community's proscriptions against readable forms of lesbian visibility, such as their shunning of women who "wear leather and sadomasochistic signifiers to social events" ("Out and About," 103).

23. Bill Short, "Up Queer Street," in *Lesbian and Gay Pride — Official Souvenir Programme*, 1993, quoted in Binnie ("Trading Places," 195). Binnie's analysis of the look of the street stops at noting that new gay bars have windows onto the street: "In these new venues, gay men are not hidden behind closed doors. Straight passers-by can look in and observe gay men, as can an increasing number of women (as these venues tend to be mixed — reflect the changing sexual landscape)" (195).

24. Benjamin Gianni and Mark Robbins, prospectus for Family Values project, 1994.

25. Similar issues might be raised in relation to Mark Robbins's subsequent "Households" project (published as *Households*), which juxtaposes photographs of domestic spaces and their inhabitants. Introduced by texts that frame this project in terms of the history of art and popular fascination with lifestyles, the project eschews claims to associate interiors with identities. Robbins states that he "hopes neither to validate nor to explode assumptions explaining identity via decor but to revel in the proof of aspiration as that proof is embedded in the array of physical terms contributing to each person's sheltering resort," as the introductory texts somewhat bafflingly conclude (aspirations to what?). The fact that many of the queer — mainly gay — residents of these spaces are pictured naked or nearly so is noted without being analyzed. For us, this fact would be the starting point of an analysis of the home as a space of sexual identity.

26. More drawings are in Weisman, *Discrimination by Design*, 172–76. Noel Phyllis Birkby's papers are in the Sophia Smith Collection at Smith College.

27. "Bachelor House" project statement at http://www.joelsandersarchitect .com/jsa.html. Sanders is further quoted from a lecture at the Museum of Contemporary Art, Chicago, 2002. For an account of a similar oral presentation of the project in 2007, describing how "Sanders created . . . a zone of privacy from outside," see http://www.cityofsound.com/blog/2007/06/postopolis_joel.html.

28. Sanders, lecture.

29. Personal correspondence (September 11, 2009).

30. For stories of specific gay men involved in restoration in San Francisco, see Fellows, *A Passion to Preserve*, 131–49.

31. Robertson was widely quoted from a June 8, 1998, episode as saying, "I would warn Orlando that you're right in the way of some serious hurricanes and

I don't think I'd be waving those flags in God's face if I were you . . . a condition like this will bring about the destruction of your nation. It'll bring about terrorist bombs; it'll bring earthquakes; tornadoes and possibly a meteor." Orlando's rainbow flags were paid for by local gay rights groups and flown from city light poles in conjunction with "Gay Days" at Disney World (http://www.skeptictank .org/hs/patrob3.htm).

32. This local history is developed in more detail in Reed, "A Third Chicago School?"

33. Interview with Edward Windhorst, October 1998.

34. Officially titled the Division Street Gateways, this project received seven professional awards, including a 1995 Distinguished Building Award from the Chicago chapter of the American Institute of Architects. Writing in *Art in America,* architectural historian and critic Franz Schulze praised the project, saying, "One could hardly imagine anything more symbolically at home on its site, or more successful in reaching the specific audience it was meant to address" ("Chicago Now," 63).

35. James B. Runnion, *Out of Town,* 1869, in Ebner, "The Result of Honest Hard Work," 177.

36. Unidentified gay man, in Weiner, "North Halsted Project." In contrast, one of the rationales for the popular support of the Puerto Rican Gates project was the belief that these structures would warn off outsiders and thus help the neighborhood resist encroaching gentrification. An antigentrification poster with the slogan "Humboldt Park no se vende" featured an image of the Gates (http://www .harakumaran.com/creativesolutions/hpnosevende/humboldtparknosevende .jpg&imgrefurl).

37. On the paradigmatic trope of urban migration, see Weston, "Get Thee to a Big City." A number of publications, including the newsletter *R.F.D.,* have challenged the incompatibility of gay and nonurban identity. This work's self-presentation as outside—and often hostile to—mainstream gay culture, however, confirms the continuing centrality of narratives of urban escape in both the history of modern gay identity and the experience of individuals who identify as gay. See, for example, Miller, *In Search of Gay America,* or Rist, *Heartlands.*

3. The Revolution Might Be Televised

1. Lipsitz focuses on how the theater "threatened a sense of authentic self-knowledge and created the psychic preconditions for the needy narcissism of consumer desire" (*Time Passages,* 7) and how television abuses this power: "Television colonizes intimate areas of human sexuality and personality, exacerbating anxieties and fears to sell more products" (18).

2. See, for example, Chauncey, *Gay New York*.

3. On *All in the Family*'s gay plots, and the ire they aroused in the Nixon White House, see Larry Gross, *Up from Visibility*, 81.

4. "Rules of Engagement," episode 4.06. The scene continues:

WILL: Yes, she did. She kept waiting for him to pop the question, and when he finally did, it was, "Do you wanna live together?" So she looked him right in the eye and said, [IMITATING RHODA] "Okay, Joe. I wanna be married."

GRACE: Wow. You will use any excuse to do a Rhoda impression.

Later in the episode, Will, again imitating Rhoda's voice, says to Grace: "Oh, Mar, we've been through so much together" (http://www.twiztv.com/scripts/willandgrace/season4/willandgrace-406). In a 2006 interview, Valerie Harper, who played Rhoda, reflects on the gay enthusiasm for her character (Hays, "Big Gay Following").

5. The enabling connections between *Rhoda* and *Will and Grace* as manifestations of minority sensibility are traced in Kera Bolonik, "Oy Gay!"

6. In 2000, Better World Advertising reported *Will and Grace*'s lead among television audiences of gay and bisexual men in the San Francisco Bay Area, among whom it earned a 36 percent share as opposed to its 6.3 percent rating in this area's population as a whole ("Surprise, Surprise," 2).

7. "*Will & Grace*," Wikipedia, accessed October 8, 2009. Other sources give the total number of Emmys as seventeen.

8. *Will and Grace* was prime among the television shows accused at a Focus on the Family conference of forwarding "the gay agenda" (Darrell Grizzle, "Fear and Trembling").

9. In contrast to the overwhelming influence of Laura Mulvey's "Visual Pleasure and Narrative Cinema," with its stated aim of destroying pleasure by analyzing it, studies of film and television rarely cite Mulvey's other writings analyzing her own viewing pleasures (most notably "Afterthoughts on 'Visual Pleasure and Narrative Cinema' Inspired by King Vidor's *Duel in the Sun*" (both in *Visual and Other Pleasures*, 14–38).

10. Schiappa, *Beyond Representational Correctness*, 68, 71, quoting Battles and Hilton-Morrow, "Gay Characters in Conventional Spaces." Battles and Hilton-Morrow continued to criticize the show as "heteronormative, despite all the critical acclaim it originally received (remember all those Emmys, Golden Globes, People's Choice, and GLAAD awards?)" ("Family, Fate").

11. Schiappa, 73, quoting Mitchell, "Producing Containment"; and Mitchell, "Rhetorically Contained."

12. In addition to Schiappa's analysis, specifically structured around responses to *Will and Grace*, the bias against pleasure instilled through the professionalization of academic critics has been analyzed by some of the most provocative

and lively writers in the humanities and social sciences. See, for instance, Pierre Bourdieu on intellectuals' need to claim an "ethical superiority" associated with "cultural capital," an impulse intensified by the confluence of popular taste and intimidating economic capital in mass entertainment *(Distinction)* or Jane Gallop's analysis of the psychic drama of criticism as an act of aggression in which the critic triumphs by debasing his/her objects of study ("Psychoanalytic Criticism").

13. Schiappa, *Beyond Representational Correctness,* 77–78, quoting Cooper.

14. Although we have expanded the range of references in this chapter occasionally beyond the first three seasons, we are not attempting an analysis of the full run of the show. At the same time, we have maintained the present-tense descriptions of the episodes we do analyze as a reflection that the show, in constant syndication, continues to function in the ways we describe.

15. Unless otherwise specified, chatroom references are to the *Will and Grace* discussion group on the NBC site at http://nbc-tvclubs.nbci.com/willandgrace/forums.

16. "Whose Mom Is It, Anyway?" episode 2.05. Except where noted, all scripts are quoted from http://www.durfee.net/will/scripts.

17. *"Will & Grace,"* Wikipedia.

18. "A Chorus Lie," episode 4.15.

19. One possible — but brief — precedent for such deployment of gay memory was the "coming out" season in the sitcom *Ellen,* but Ellen's obliviousness to — and outright denial of — subcultural allusions during the protracted buildup to the coming out (as described by Gross, *Up from Visibility,* 157–58, and Walters, *All the Rage,* 83) left little time for their development before the show's cancellation. What Walters describes as the "snatches of gay life" in the last shows of the season (88–90) did manifest many of the dynamics we find in *Will and Grace,* however.

20. This thread is discussed in note 23.

21. "Love Plus One," episode 3.06.

22. "Brothers, a Love Story," episode 3.13.

23. In response to the thread, "Do you think the reason everyone loves Jack so much is because he is stereotypically gay and Will acts like he's straight? Do you think it will help when Will gets a boyfriend?" came replies such as, "I would definitely love to see him with a partner or significant other and would not mind at all if they called on me!" and "I would love to see Will play a more gay role, more real to life. Yes, actually dating and relationship issues with other gay men would be a plus." Although viewers can imagine Will with a "boyfriend or significant other" or celibate, they reject the idea that Will should have serial partners. As one viewer put it, "He does deserve someone in his life. But I do not think

they should put him around with all kinds of guys. Will is usually the one with emotional attachments and I think to have this with all the guys would go against his character."

24. Recognition of this range drove the inclusion of Jack as a second gay character during the show's initial development, according to Max Mutchnik, one of the show's creators: "When we first wrote the pilot they were one character" (Kirby, "The Boys," 33).

25. "Alice Doesn't Live Here Anymore," episode 3.20.

26. "Love Plus One," episode 3.06.

27. "Coffee and Commitment," episode 3.10.

28. "Ben? Her?" episode 2.23. That straight women characters prove as adept at camp as gay men is not surprising, given the history of camp, which often arose from figures — Bette Davis or Mae West, for example — who appealed to female and gay male viewers because of similar traits of endurance, self-assertion, and erotic inventiveness. In response to the thread "Which character do you relate to the best? Why?" one posting reads, "Karen's the woman I'd want to be! . . . To be able to completely overlook all my MANY faults and just roast everyone I see. That takes guts and quite a bit of confidence."

29. "Fear and Clothing," episode 3.02.

30. "Love Plus One," episode 3.06.

31. David Kohan, quoted in Kirby, 33. Gay novelist Andrew Holleran, characterizing Karen as "a cross between Leona Helmsley, Lorena Bobbitt, Jacqueline Susann, Mother Goddam, and Margo Channing," claims her as, "Let's face it — the only really gay character on the whole sitcom: the straight woman." For Holleran, gay identification with Karen is a function of a nostalgic and collective yearning arising from strong cultural memory: "We miss Paul Lynde. We miss Wayland Flowers and Madame. We miss Bette Davis. We even miss the Golden Girls" ("Alpha Queen").

32. Howard Buford, president of the advertising agency behind the campaign to market *Queer as Folk,* described his premise: "It's relevant to a broader audience if you convince them the show is an authentic slice of gay and lesbian life" (in Elliot, "Advertising"). Mainstream television critics bought this claim, rehearsing clichés of the "hard-hitting" *Queer as Folk* as praiseworthy for the realistic "fullness of the characters" in contrast to shows like *Will and Grace,* and quoting *Queer as Folk*'s executive producer on the need "to be honest" (in Johnson, "'Quare' Studies").

33. The NBC chatroom devoted to the show reveals that Jack and Karen's relationship at least equals — and threatens to overwhelm — the draw of the show's original couple. Discussion threads "*Will & Grace* or Jack & Karen?" and "Who's funnier Will and Grace or Jack and Karen" elicited only responses favoring Jack

and Karen, with the exception of two participants who tactfully urged that the two pairs were equally funny. See also the discussion thread "Who loved that episode?"

34. "To Serve and Disinfect," episode 2.07.

35. "I Never Promised You an Olive Garden," episode 2.3. The power of this image of camp mentorship is registered in such chatroom postings as "My favorite episode was when Jack came to the rescue of the young boy in the school hallway. We all could have used a Jack when we were that age!" (http://htmlgear.lycos.com).

36. Jack's attitude toward his "theft"—acknowledging but unconcerned—implies a queer critique of the dominant culture's valorization of individuality in several ways. First, mainstream culture grants married heterosexuals a notion of collective property that it denies gay couples; if Jack and Bjorn were straight and married, the fact that this product was Bjorn's idea would be less troubling. Second, Jack reveals the fallacy behind presumptions that capitalism or the law represent the triumph of "originality": the jingles he recycles in his performance are attractive because they are repeated in commercials, and the legal case the investors threaten Jack with would be built upon a derivative notion of precedent.

37. For a strong critique of niche marketing, see Chasin, *Selling Out*, 101–43; Chasin acknowledges "leaving aside" issues of gay and lesbian "cultural expression, taste, subjectivity, and lifestyle" (xx). For the argument that *Will and Grace*, along with other American television and film, presents assimilationist queer characters that leave mainstream viewers' prejudices unchallenged, see Keller, *Queer (Un)Friendly Film*.

38. This case has been made particularly strongly for the niche-marketed physique magazines of the 1950s and 1960s. These offered men "membership" (as subscriptions were called) in a community that valued homoeroticism along with other pleasures of the body and challenged authoritative legal and medical definitions of normality and probity, creating a far closer precedent to the activist forms of gay community that emerged in the late 1960s than the earnestly assimilationist political magazines. Though the circulation of the physique magazines was hundreds of times greater than that of the political periodicals, political histories of the gay movement have been blinded to their influence by assumptions of the apolitical nature of mass culture to the extent of ignoring and denying the political commentary that accompanied the beefcake pictures (Nealon, *Foundlings*, 99–139).

39. Until recently, the most enabling queer scholarship on film and television explicated depictions of homosexuality not named as such in mainstream film and television. The chapter "The Way We Weren't" in Vito Russo's pioneering *The Celluloid Closet* set a standard for this kind of work; other valuable examples include Richard Dyer, *The Matter of Images*.

40. A partial catalog might include the African American girl Jack competes with on e-Bay, a trick named Mipanko and his unnamed father, a delivery boy, a temperance-oriented soccer mom, an INS officer, a crowd of "recovering" gays and lesbians, Martina Navratilova, a crew of ballet-dancing cater-waiters, a gay-acting heterosexual named Scott, a weeping woman in a bar, and a porn director.

41. "Whose Mom Is It, Anyway," episode 2.05.

42. "Gypsies, Tramps and Weed," episode 3.7.

43. Thread: "Which character do you relate to the best? Why?"

44. This validation has been a long time coming, as television lags behind so-cial trends registered in well-known sociological studies since the 1970s (Nahas and Turley, *The New Couple*).

45. In addition to these responses to the thread "Are any guys/girls in a 'Will and Grace' relationship??" other posters identify with the Karen–Jack duo. One woman posted, "My friend Joel is my 'Just Jack.' He's every girl's best friend" (thread: *Will & Grace* or Jack & Karen). Another female viewer acknowledged, "While watching *Will & Grace*, I never wanted to be a gay man so badly." Not surprisingly, she identifies especially with Jack: "I love Jack (sounds corny but true)!!!!!!" (http://htmlgear.lycos.com). Another female viewer writes, "I'd have to say I'm a lot like Jack. Which is kinda sad because I'm a 13 year old female and he's a 30 year old gay guy. Ah, it doesn't bother me, but he acts like I do in so many ways (which may be why I love him so much) he could maybe even pass for my brother or some-thing"—the "or something" here reveals the glimmer in this young viewer's mind of a possibility for a relationship outside the norms of the nuclear family (thread: "Which character do you relate to the best? Why?"). The fluidity of identifications fostered by *Will and Grace* is truly queer and clearly contradicts assumptions that all gay people identify with "positive images" like the one presented by the charac-ter of Will or that only gay men benefit from the forms of identification and self-esteem arising from gay-identified cultural forms like camp and cruising.

46. http://htmlgear.lycos.com.

47. Threads: "Is it the gay thing, or do we really like the show?" and "Which character do you relate to the best? Why?"

48. This point is made repeatedly in the chatrooms: one participant charac-terizes *Will and Grace* as "show[ing] two gay men who only kiss and have sex with women. . . . I appreciate *Will & Grace*. I'd just appreciate it more if they didn't shy away from being gay" (thread: "Gay Representation on TV"); see also thread "Kiss Tally."

49. "Alice Doesn't Live Here Anymore," episode 3.20.

50. "*Will & Grace*," Wikipedia.

51. In what seems intended as a gracious conclusion, Bianco's churlish review ends with, "It is possible to watch *Will* and think gay men are abnormal—but it is

not possible to watch it and think gay men accept that definition, which had been the common cultural assumption. *Will* took people who were once seen only as targets of jokes or objects of pity and let them just be people. That may be accomplishment enough." Blind to any intimation of the value of subculture, this writer implies that valid personhood requires the rejection of "abnormality."

52. "The Finale," episode 8.23.

53. "Sons and Lovers," episode 3.22.

4. Queer Theory Is Burning

1. We date the first wave in queer theory as running between Eve Kosofsky Sedgwick's 1985 *Between Men* and Leo Bersani's 1995 *Homos,* although Sedgwick was in many ways uncharacteristic of the first wave of queer theory, particularly in her consistent acknowledgment of the relationship between contemporary sexual cultures, AIDS, and gay and lesbian liberation politics. Above all, Sedgwick, whose concept of "reparative reading" is important to our analysis here, resisted both the abstraction of sexuality and what Michael Snediker calls "queer pessimism": the "suspiciously routinized" attachment to concepts such as "melancholy, self-shattering, shame, the death drive" (*Queer Optimism,* 4). On queer pessimism in the work of Judith Butler and Leo Bersani, and Eve Sedgwick's resistances to it, see Snediker, 1–15.

2. Our characterization of first-wave queer theory rests on its self-presentation as a corrective to prevailing ideas of "gay" and "lesbian" identity. We are not alone in seeking to reexamine queer theory's relation to these earlier political and critical constructions of minority sexuality or in recognizing retrospectively the connections between first-wave queer theory and AIDS. Annamarie Jagose, in *Queer Theory: An Introduction,* connects queer theory with the pre-AIDS homophile, lesbian feminist, and gay liberation movements. The relationship between queer theory and AIDS is recognized in the collective—albeit garbled—knowledge represented by Wikipedia. The Wikipedia entry on "queer theory" is one of the few places where queer theory is directly associated with AIDS. The entry reports, "Much of queer theory developed out of a response to the AIDS crisis, which promoted a renewal of radical activism, and the growing homophobia brought about by public responses to AIDS. Queer theory became occupied in part with what effects—put into circulation around the AIDS epidemic—necessitated and nurtured new forms of political organization, education, and theorizing in 'queer'" [sic] (accessed April 12, 2011). Despite the important theorists who did focus on AIDS and its effects, however, much of what came to be canonized as "queer theory" was not "occupied" with these issues.

3. The *Diagnostic and Statistical Manual of Mental Disorders*, 4th ed., describes the "essential features" of post-traumatic stress disorder as "the development of characteristic symptoms following exposure to an extreme traumatic stress or involving direct personal experience of an event that involves actual or threatened death or serious injury, or other threat to one's physical integrity; or witnessing an event that involves death, injury, or a threat to the physical integrity of another person; or learning about unexpected or violent death, serious harm, or threat of death or injury experienced by a family member or other close associate (Criterion A1). The person's response to the event must involve intense fear, helplessness, or horror (or in children, the response must involve disorganized or agitated behavior) (Criterion A2). The characteristic symptoms resulting from the exposure to the extreme trauma include persistent re-experiencing of the traumatic event (Criterion B), persistent avoidance of stimuli associated with the trauma and numbing of general responsiveness (Criterion C), and persistent symptoms of increased arousal (Criterion D)" (424).

The horrifying encounter with death and dying on an unprecedented scale, combined with the anxiety of often not knowing one's own HIV status, the fear of losing one's home or job or family due to discrimination, the persistent frustration of inadequate — or no — health care, the rage at press and popular cultural misrepresentations, and the disorientating perception that AIDS is an *unreal* phenomenon, rendered invisible in mainstream culture while hypervisible to those responding to its ravages, qualify AIDS as a trauma by the DSM definition, several times over.

4. Trauma theorist Dominick LaCapra argues, "Modern society is characterized by a dearth of social processes, including ritual processes, which assist individuals during major transformations in life such as marriage, birth, or death" (*Writing History, Writing Trauma*, 213). Where LaCapra sees "general tendencies toward the evacuation of engaging collective forms and rituals" (213), we point to specific inequities in "modern society's" distribution of ritual. There are plenty of rituals surrounding the heteronormative "major transformations" of marriage and birth, an abundance that is particularly striking in comparison to the paucity and poverty of rituals to mark the death of people with AIDS and the sexual cultures they created.

5. Caruth describes how that "threat is recognized as such by the mind *one moment too late*. The shock of the mind's relation to the threat of death is thus not the direct experience of the threat but precisely the *missing* of this experience, the fact that, not being experienced *in time*, it has not yet been fully known" (*Unclaimed Experience*, 62). The "historical power of the trauma is not just that the experience is repeated after its forgetting," therefore, "but that it is only in and through its inherent forgetting that it is first experienced at all" (17).

6. A significant exception to this normalizing treatment of trauma can be found in Ann Cvetkovich's *An Archive of Feelings,* which connects trauma, memory, and AIDS in a spirit of activism. For Cvetkovich, trauma is "a name for experiences of socially situated political violence" (3). A queer treatment of such experiences, she argues, would neither "pathologize it" nor "seize control over it from the medical experts," but would "forge creative responses to it that far outstrip even the most utopian of therapeutic and political solutions" (3). Cvetkovich is not "willing to accept a desexualized or sanitized version of queer culture as the price of inclusion within the national public sphere"; instead, she "wanted the sexual cultures that AIDS threatened to be acknowledged as both an achievement and a potential loss" (5). Writing, "My desire, forged from the urgency of death, has been to keep the history of AIDS activism alive and part of the present" (6), Cvetkovich establishes her "archive" as a valuable model of memory for queer theory.

7. On Solanas and Gornick, see Reed, *Art and Homosexuality,* 175.

8. Halberstam misspells Eisenman's name as Eiseman. Eisenman's highly successful career has been accompanied by numerous statements in which she rejects the label of "lesbian artist" and even "female artist," because, as a quotation prominently featured on her New York gallery's Web site puts it, "I don't see myself as being in a combative stance" (http://www.artseensoho.com/Art/ TILTON/eisenman96/ei1 [accessed July 27, 2006]). On Eisenman, see Reed, *Art and Homosexuality,* 242–44.

5. Remembering a New Queer Politics

1. Vito Russo discusses the significance of this line in *The Celluloid Closet* (65).

2. Neil Bartlett's *Who Was That Man?* offers an evocative counterexample, not written by a historian.

3. Eng and Kazanjian offer an astute analysis of the relation between loss and ideals in Agamben: "Agamben's medieval melancholia materializes the ghostly remains of an unrealized or idealized potential—the unreal image of an unobtainable object that never was and hence was never lost. Indeed, it is precisely by imagining such a space for the remains of the past that those remains can emerge as constricting forces or motivating ideals" (*Loss,* 13).

4. Information on the NAMES Project Quilt is culled from http://www .aidsquilt.org and Ruskin, *The Quilt,* 9.

5. Andrew McNamara ("Illegible Echoes") understands Gonzalez-Torres's temporal play in terms of Walter Benjamin's conception of "remembrance" as a counterforce to official history, giving voice to what has been forgotten or repressed in the success stories of history. Quoting Rainer Rochlitz's account (in

The Disenchantment of Art) of Benjamin's theories of memory as "the irritant that disrupts historical narratives presuming the untrammeled success or superiority of the present" through which "the injustices of the past can haunt the present," McNamara sets Gonzalez-Torres's work in the context of art's ethical function of saving (again quoting Rochlitz) "from mutism and forgetting certain irreplaceable experiences to which society assigns no other rightful place."

For McNamara, however, this process remains locked in the history of art. The "tradition" that Gonzalez-Torres saves is about art "such as minimalism" and "earlier modernist practices such as Russian Constructivism and Dada." Despite his intriguing focus on memory and recuperation, McNamara follows the many other art historians who have "overwhelmingly concentrated" on placing Gonzalez-Torres's work in relation to the history of minimalism (Watney, *Imagine Hope,* 161)—a tendency encouraged by the foundation that controls posthumous rights to reproduce his art (Moore, *Beyond Shame,* 171). McNamara opens his argument by distancing Gonzalez-Torres from traditions associated with gay identity, claiming, "Gonzalez-Torres largely distanced himself from identity politics and from any attempt to determine a reading of his work based upon him being gay or Hispanic." The quotations from the artist that McNamara adduces to support this claim, however, address only his resistance to being confined to a Hispanic identity that would seem to preclude legitimate connection to a list of non-Hispanics headed by Gertrude Stein. In fact, in the interview from which these quotations are taken, the artist prefaces his remarks about his love of reading with, "It's a queer thing, I mean, at least from my background" (in Bartman et al., *Between Artists,* 86), and he distances himself from attempts to attribute to him any sense of being mentored by minimalists (87–88). We do not doubt that Gonzalez-Torres was a sophisticated artist well versed in histories of avant-garde artistic practice. We do contest, however, the disciplinary boundary policing that repeatedly asserts an evolutionary history of art as the primary focus of art criticism and history (on this tendency more broadly, see Reed, *Art and Homosexuality,* 242–48).

6. We follow Wäspe in treating both the Photostats and the artist's room-scale bands of similar texts as "portraits": "biographic combinations [that] consist of the most important events in the life of a person (or institution)" ("Private and Public," 19). The Felix Gonzalez-Torres Foundation reserves the term "portrait" for the room-scale pieces.

7. This self-portrait, *"Untitled,"* is now jointly owned by the Art Institute of Chicago and the San Francisco Museum of Modern Art.

8. "Sexual theatre" is quoted from http://www.delmashowe.com/stationsAlt.html.

9. Personal correspondence, August 16, 2010.

10. "As with minor literatures," Berlant writes, "minor intimacies have been forced to develop aesthetics of the extreme to push these spaces into being by way of small and grand gestures" ("Intimacy," 5–6).

11. Jon Bastian, in "Chuck & Buck (2000)," describes the film as "both innocently sappy and terribly creepy." A. O. Scott calls it "an intimate, slightly creepy, often disturbing look at loneliness and need" ("'Chuck and Buck'").

12. In *The Psychic Life of Power*, Judith Butler writes, "If we accept the notion that heterosexuality naturalizes itself by insisting on the radical otherness of homosexuality, then heterosexual identity is purchased through a melancholic incorporation of the love that it disavows: the man who insists upon the coherence of his heterosexuality will claim that he never loved another man, and hence never lost another man. That love, that attachment becomes subject to a double disavowal, a never having loved, and never having lost. This 'never-never' thus founds the heterosexual subject, as it were; it is an identity based upon the refusal to avow an attachment and, hence, the refusal to grieve" (139–40).

13. The lost object of melancholic longing might, Freud wrote, be found among those "in his near neighbourhood" ("Mourning and Melancholia," 170).

14. Thanks to Jonathan Walz for pointing out the important symbolism of the theater's name.

15. This portrait of Buck, as James Keller notes, exaggerates the frequent unkind characterizations of gay men "as irresponsible and sexually and socially under-developed" (*Queer (Un)Friendly Film*, 193).

16. Bordowitz, *The AIDS Crisis Is Ridiculous*, xix, quoted in Juhasz, "Video Remains," 326.

BIBLIOGRAPHY

Agamben, Giorgio. *The Coming Community: Theory out of Bounds.* 1990. Trans. Michael Hardt. Minneapolis: University of Minnesota Press, 1993.

———. *Infancy and History: On the Destruction of Experience.* 1978. Trans. Liz Heron. London: Verso, 1993.

———. *Stanzas: Word and Phantasm in Western Culture.* 1977. Trans. Ronald L. Martinez. Minneapolis: University of Minnesota Press, 1993.

Ahmed, Sara. *Queer Phenomenology: Orientations, Objects, Others.* Durham, N.C.: Duke University Press, 2006.

Altman, Dennis. "Liberation: Toward the Polymorphous." 1971. In Escoffier, *Sexual Revolution,* 616–42.

Anderson, Benedict R. *Imagined Communities: Reflections on the Origin and Spread of Nationalism.* New York: Verso, 1983.

Anonymous. "Cocksucker." 1971. In Escoffier, *Sexual Revolution,* 513–15.

Appadurai, Arjun. *Modernity at Large: Cultural Dimensions of Globalization.* Minneapolis: University of Minnesota Press, 1996.

Bal, Mieke, Jonathan Crewe, and Leo Spitzer, eds. *Acts of Memory: Cultural Recall in the Present.* Hanover, N.H.: University Press of New England, 1999.

Banchero, Stephanie. "City Offers Toned-Down North Halsted Plan." *Chicago Tribune,* November 13, 1997, 2C1.

———. "Gay Theme Toned Down in Halsted St. Plan." *Chicago Tribune,* November 2, 1997, 4C4.

Bartlett, Neil. *Who Was That Man? A Gift for Mr. Oscar Wilde.* London: Serpent's Tail, 1988.

Bartman, William, Lucinda Barnes, Miyoshi Barosh, Rodney Sappington, and Dave Hickey, eds. *Between Artists: Twelve Contemporary American Artists Interview Twelve Contemporary American Artists.* Los Angeles: ART Press, 1996.

Bastian, Jon. "Chuck & Buck (2000)." http://www.filmmonthly.com/video_and_dvd/chuck_and_buck.html.

Battles, Kathleen, and Wendy Hilton-Morrow. "Family, Fate and the Finale of *Will and Grace.*" *Flow-TV,* posted July 7, 2006. http://flowtv.org.

———. "Gay Characters in Conventional Spaces: *Will & Grace* and the Situation Comedy Genre." *Critical Studies in Media Communication* 19 (2002): 87–105.

Bell, David. "One-Handed Geographies: An Archeology of Public Sex." In Ingram, Bouthillette, and Retter, *Queers in Space,* 81–87.

Bell, David, and Gill Valentine, eds. *Mapping Desire: Geographies of Sexuality.* New York: Routledge, 1995.

Berlant, Lauren. "Intimacy: A Special Issue." In *Intimacy,* ed. Lauren Berlant, 3–8. Chicago: University of Chicago Press, 2000.

Berlant, Lauren, and Michael Warner. "Sex in Public." *Critical Inquiry* 24, no. 2 (Winter 1998): 547–66.

Bersani, Leo. *Homos.* Cambridge, Mass.: Harvard University Press, 1996.

———. "Is the Rectum a Grave?" *October* 43 (1987): 197–222.

Betsky, Aaron. *Queer Space: Architecture and Same-Sex Desire.* New York: William Morrow, 1997.

Bianco, Robert. "So Who, Exactly, Were Those People?" *USA Today,* May 18, 2006. http://www.usatoday.com/life/television/reviews/2006-05-17-willgracereview.

Binnie, Jon. "Trading Places: Consumption, Sexuality and the Production of Queer Space." In Bell and Valentine, *Mapping Desire,* 182–99.

Birkby, Phyllis. "Herspace." *Heresies* 11 (1981): 28–29.

Birkby, Noel Phyllis, and Leslie Kanes Weisman. "A Woman Built Environment: Constructive Fantasies." *Quest: A Feminist Quarterly* 2, no. 1 (Summer 1975): 7–18.

Bolonik, Kera. "Oy Gay!" *The Nation,* November 17, 2003.

Bordowitz, Gregg. *The AIDS Crisis Is Ridiculous and Other Writings: 1986–2003,* ed. James Meyer. Cambridge, Mass.: MIT Press, 2004.

Bourdieu, Pierre. *Distinction: A Social Critique of the Judgment of Taste.* Trans. Richard Nice. Cambridge, Mass.: Harvard University Press, 1984.

Boyce, David B. "The Making of *Gay Liberation* (the Statue)." *Harvard Gay and Lesbian Review* 4, no. 2 (Spring 1997): 11–13.

Bronski, Michael. "Reel Politick." *Z*, September 1992, 73–75.

Brown, Bill. "Thing Theory." *Critical Inquiry* 28 (Autumn 2001): 1–16.

Burlein, Ann. "Countermemory on the Right: The Case of Focus on the Family." In Bal, Crewe, and Spitzer, *Acts of Memory*, 208–17.

Burston, Paul. "Just a Gigolo? Narcissism, Nellyism, and the 'New Man' Theme." In *A Queer Romance: Lesbians, Gay Men and Popular Culture*, ed. Paul Burston and Colin Richardson, 120–32. London: Routledge, 1995.

Butler, Connie. "Queer Space." *Art + Text* 49 (September 1994): 83–84.

Butler, Judith. *The Psychic Life of Power: Theories in Subjection*. Stanford, Calif.: Stanford University Press, 1997.

Byrne, Dennis. "Everybody on Board Halsted St. Express." *Chicago Sun-Times* August 17, 1997, 13

Califia, Pat. "A Secret Side of Lesbian Sexuality." 1979. In Escoffier, *Sexual Revolution*, 527–37.

Caruth, Cathy. *Unclaimed Experience: Trauma, Narrative, and History*. Baltimore, Md.: Johns Hopkins University Press, 1996.

Castells, Manuel. *The City and the Grassroots: A Cross-Cultural Theory of Urban Social Movements*. Berkeley: University of California Press, 1983.

Castiglia, Christopher. *Interior States*. Durham, N.C.: Duke University Press, 2008.

———. "Sex Panics, Sex Publics, Sex Memories." *boundary 2* 27, no. 2 (2000): 149–75.

Chase, John. *Exterior Decoration: Hollywood's Inside-out Houses*. Los Angeles: Hennessey and Ingalls, 1982.

Chasin, Alexandra. *Selling Out: The Gay and Lesbian Movement Goes to Market*. New York: St. Martin's Press, 2000.

Chater, David. "Viewing Guide," *Times* (London), June 11, 2004, T2, 24.

Chauncey, George. *Gay New York*. New York: Basic, 1995.

———. "'Privacy Could Only Be Had in Public': Gay Uses of the Streets." In Sanders, *Stud*, 224–60.

Chuck & Buck. Dir. Miguel Arteta. Perf. Mike White, Chris Weitz, Paul Weitz. Artisan Entertainment, 2000.

Cooper, Evan. "Decoding *Will & Grace*: Mass Audience Reception of a Popular Network Situation Comedy." *Sociological Perspectives* 46 (2003): 513–33.

Crain, Caleb. "Pleasure Principles: Queer Theorists and Gay Journalists Wrestle Over the Politics of Sex." *Lingua Franca* (October 1997): 26–37.

Crimp, Douglas. *Melancholia and Moralism: Essays on AIDS and Queer Politics*. Cambridge, Mass.: MIT Press, 2002.

———. "Mourning and Militancy." In Crimp, *Melancholia and Moralism*, 125–46.

Crout, Durham. "Wasting Architecture." *Vulvamorphia*, special issue of *Lusitania* 6 (1994): 13–22.

Cvetkovich, Ann. *An Archive of Feelings: Trauma, Sexuality, and Lesbian Public Cultures.* Durham, N.C.: Duke University Press, 2003.

Dean, Tim. "The Antisocial Homosexual." *PMLA* 21, no. 3 (May 2006): 826–28.

———. *Unlimited Intimacy: Reflections on the Subculture of Barebacking.* Chicago: University of Chicago Press, 2009.

D'Emilio, John. "Capitalism and Gay Identity." In *Powers of Desire: The Politics of Sexuality,* ed. Ann Snitow, Christine Stansell, and Sharon Thompson, 100–113. New York: Monthly Review Press, 1983.

Demos, John. "Oedipus and America: Historical Perspectives on the Reception of Psychoanalysis in the United States." 1978. In *Inventing the Psychological: Toward a Cultural History of Emotional Life in America,* ed. Joel Pfister and Nancy Schnog, 63–78. New Haven: Yale University Press, 1997.

Désert, Jean-Ulrick. "Queer Space." In Ingram, Bouthillette, and Retter, *Queers in Space,* 17–26.

Diagnostic and Statistical Manual of Mental Disorders, 4th ed. Washington, D.C.: American Psychiatric Association, 1994.

Doyle, Brian. "The Love Songs of Jacob Israel de Haan." *Gay & Lesbian Review Worldwide* 13, no. 5 (September–October, 2006): 3536.

Doyle, Vincent. "'But Joan! You're My Daughter!' The Gay and Lesbian Alliance Against Defamation and the Politics of Amnesia." *Radical History Review* 100 (Winter 2008): 209–21.

Dubrow, Gail Lee. "Blazing Trails with Pink Triangles and Rainbow Flags: Improving the Preservation and Interpretation of Gay and Lesbian Heritage." In *Restoring Women's History through Historic Preservation,* ed. Gail Lee Dubrow and Jennifer B. Goodman, 281. Baltimore, Md.: Johns Hopkins University Press, 2003.

Dyer, Richard. *The Matter of Images: Essays on Representations.* London: Routledge, 1993.

Ebner, Michael H. "The Result of Honest Hard Work: Creating a Suburban Ethos for Evanston." In *A Wild Kind of Boldness: The Chicago History Reader,* ed. Rosemary K. Adams, 176–89. Chicago: Chicago Historical Society, 1998.

Edelman, Lee. "Antagonism, Negativity, and the Subject of Queer Theory." *PMLA* 21, no. 3 (May 2006): 821–23.

———. "Men's Room." in Sanders, *Stud,* 152–61.

———. *No Future: Queer Theory and the Death Drive.* Durham, N.C.: Duke University Press, 2004.

Elger, Dietmar. "Catalogue Raisonné." Vol. 2. of *Felix Gonzalez-Torres.*

Elliot, Stuart. "Advertising." *New York Times,* November 28, 2000.

Eng, David, and David Kazanjian. *Loss: The Politics of Mourning.* Berkeley: University of California Press, 2003.

Engelbrecht, P. J. "North Halsted Streetscape Plans 'Set' Says CDOT Commish," *Outlines* November 26, 1997. http://www.outlineschicago.com/archives/current/archives/112697/halsted.

Epstein, Steven. "Gay Politics, Ethnic Identity: The Limits of Social Constructionism." 1987. In *Unfinished Business: Twenty Years of Socialist Review,* ed. Socialist Review, 69–91. London: Verso, 1991.

Escoffier, Jeffrey, ed. *Sexual Revolution.* New York: Thunder's Mouth, 2003.

Featherstone, Mike. "Global and Local Cultures." In *Mapping the Futures: Local Cultures, Global Change,* ed. Jon Bird, Barry Curtis, Tim Putnam, George Robertson, and Lisa Tickner, 169–87. London: Routledge, 1993.

Felix Gonzalez-Torres. 2 vols. New York: Distributed Art Publishers, 1997.

Fellows, Will. *A Passion to Preserve: Gay Men as Keepers of Culture.* Madison: University of Wisconsin Press, 2004,

Fischhoff, Baruch. "An Early History of Hindsight Research." *Social Cognition* 25, no. 1 (2007): 10–13.

Foucault, Michel. "Film and Popular Memory." 1974. Trans. Martin Jordan. In Lotringer, *Foucault Live,* 89–106.

——. "Friendship as a Way of Life." 1981. Trans. John Johnston. In Lotringer, *Foucault Live,* 203–9.

——. *The History of Sexuality, Volume 3: The Care of the Self.* Trans. Robert Hurley. New York: Random House, 1988.

——. "Nietzsche, Genealogy, History." 1971. In *Language, Counter-Memory, Practice: Selected Essays and Interviews by Michel Foucault,* ed. Donald F. Bouchard, trans. Donald F. Bouchard and Sherry Simon, 139–64. Ithaca, N.Y.: Cornell University Press, 1977.

——. "Sexual Choice, Sexual Act." 1982. Trans. James O'Higgins. In Lotringer, *Foucault Live,* 211–31.

Freeman, Elizabeth. "Introduction: Theorizing Queer Temporalities: a Roundtable Discussion." *GLQ* 13, no. 2–3 (2007): 159–76.

——. "Packing History, Count(er)ing Generations." *New Literary History* 31 (2000): 727–44.

——. "Turn the Beat Around: Sadomasochism, Temporality, History." *differences: a journal of feminist cultural studies* 19, no. 1 (2008): 32–70.

Freud, Sigmund. "Mourning and Melancholia." In *General Psychological Theory,* 164–79. New York: Simon and Schuster, 1991.

Friedman, Alice T. *Women and the Making of the Modern House: A Social and Architectural History.* New York: Harry N. Abrams, 1998.

Frisch, Suzy. "Gay-Pride Theme on Halsted Is Protested." *Chicago Tribune*, September 4, 1997, 2C1.

Gallop, Jane. "Psychoanalytic Criticism: Some Intimate Questions." *Art in America* 72 (November 1984): 9–15.

Gianni, Benjamin, Scott Weir, Eve Kosofsky Sedgwick, and Michael Moon. "Queerying (Single Family) Space." *Sites* 26 (1995): 54–57.

"GLAAD Study Reveals Slow But Steady Increase in Numbers of LGBT Characters for 2009–2010 Broadcast TV Season." News release, October 1, 2009. http://www.glaad.org.

Gooch, Brad. *The Golden Age of Promiscuity*. New York: Knopf, 1996.

Grizzle, Darrell. "Fear and Trembling at an Ex-Gay Confab." *Gay and Lesbian Review Worldwide* (January/February 2002). http://www.dialogweb.com/cgi/document.

Gross, Larry. *Up from Visibility: Lesbians, Gay Men, and the Media in America.* New York: Columbia University Press, 2001.

Gurganus, Allan. "Preservation News." 1994. In *The Practical Heart: Four Novellas*, 73–118. New York: Alfred A. Knopf, 2001.

Halberstam, Judith. *In a Queer Time and Place: Transgender Bodies, Subcultural Lives.* New York: New York University Press, 2005.

———. "The Politics of Negativity in Recent Queer Theory." *PMLA* 121, no. 3 (May 2006): 823–25.

Halley, Janet, and Andrew Parker, eds. *After Sex? On Writing since Queer Theory.* Special issue of *South Atlantic Quarterly* 106, no. 3 (Summer 2007).

Halperin, David. *Saint Foucault: Towards a Gay Hagiography.* New York: Oxford University Press, 1995.

Hay, Harry. *Radically Gay: Gay Liberation in the Words of Its Founder.* Ed. Will Roscoe. Boston: Beacon, 1996.

Hays, Matthew. "Big Gay Following." *Advocate* 31 (January 2006). http://www.thefreelibrary.com.

Heidemann, Jason A. "Sonny and Sheer." *Time Out Chicago* 237 (September 10–16, 2009). http://chicago.timeout.com/articles/gay/78306/doug-ischar-at-golden-gallery-photography.

Holleran, Andrew. *Ground Zero.* New York: New American Library, 1988.

———. "The Alpha Queen." *Gay & Lesbian Review* 7, no. 3 (Summer 2000).

Hollibaugh, Amber, and Cherríe Moraga. "What We're Rollin' Around in Bed With." 1981. In Escoffier, *Sexual Revolution*, 538–52.

Humphrey, Laud. *Tearoom Trade.* Chicago: Aldine, 1975.

Huyssen, Andreas. *Present Pasts: Urban Palimpsests and the Politics of Memory.* Stanford, Calif.: Stanford University Press, 2003.

————. "Resistance to Memory: The Uses and Abuses of Public Forgetting." In *Globalizing Critical Theory*, ed. Max Pensky, 165–84. London: Rowan and Littlefield, 2005.

Ingram, Gordon Brent, Anne-Marie Bouthillette, and Yolanda Retter, eds. *Queers in Space: Communities, Public Places, Sites of Resistance*. Seattle: Bay Press, 1997.

Jagose, Annamarie. *Queer Theory: An Introduction*. New York: New York University Press, 1997.

Jencks, Charles. *Daydream Houses of Los Angeles*. New York: Rizzoli, 1978.

————. "Genealogy of Post-Modern Architecture," *Architectural Design* 47 (April 1977): 269–71.

————. *The Language of Post-Modern Architecture*. New York: Rizzoli, 1977.

Johnson, E. Patrick. "'Quare' Studies, or (Almost) Everything I Know about Queer Studies I Learned from My Grandmother." In *Black Queer Studies*, ed. E. Patrick Johnson and Mae G. Henderson, 124–59. Durham, N.C.: Duke University Press, 2005.

Johnson, Steve. "On Television: On the Gaydar." *Chicago Tribune*, November 30, 2000.

Johnston, Jill. "The Myth of the Myth of the Vaginal Orgasm." 1973. In Escoffier, *Sexual Revolution*, 504–12.

Judt, Tony. *Reappraisals: Reflections on the Forgotten Twentieth Century*. New York: Penguin, 2008.

Juhasz, Alexandra. "Video Remains: Nostalgia, Technology, and Queer Archive Activism." *GLQ* 12, no. 2 (2006): 319–28.

Keller, James R. *Queer (Un)Friendly Film and Television*. Jefferson, N.C.: McFarland, 2002.

Kimmelman, Michael. "Sculpture, Sculpture Everywhere." *New York Times*, July 31, 1992, accessed at http://www.nytimes.com.

Kirby, David. "The Boys in the Writers' Room." *New York Times* June 17, 2001, K23, 33.

Koenders, Pieter. *Het Homomonument/The Homomonument*. Amsterdam: Stichting Homomonument, 1987.

Kraft, Ronald. "This Gay House." *The Advocate* 24 (August 1993): 56–59.

Kramer, Hilton. *The Revenge of the Philistines: Art and Culture 1972–1984*. London: Secker and Warburg, 1985.

LaCapra, Dominick. *Writing History, Writing Trauma*. Baltimore, Md.: Johns Hopkins University Press, 2001.

Lanigan-Schmidt, Thomas. "Mother Stonewall and the Golden Rats." Handwritten flyer. 1992. New York Public Library, Manuscripts and Archives Division, Martin B. Duberman Papers.

Lipsitz, George. *Time Passages: Collective Memory and American Popular Culture.* Minneapolis: University of Minnesota Press, 1990.

Lipton, Lawrence. From *The Erotic Revolution.* 1965. In Escoffier, *Sexual Revolution,* 175–85.

Locke, John. *An Essay concerning Human Understanding.* 1690. In *Theories of Memory: A Reader,* ed. Michael Rossington and Anne Whitehead, 75–79. Baltimore, Md.: Johns Hopkins University Press, 2007.

Lorde, Audre. "Uses of the Erotic: The Erotics of Power." 1978. In Escoffier, *Sexual Revolution,* 166–74.

Lotringer, Sylvère, ed. *Foucault Live (Interviews, 1966–84).* New York: Semiotext(e), 1989.

Love, Heather. *Feeling Backward: Loss and the Politics of Queer History.* Cambridge, Mass.: Harvard University Press, 2008.

Lucey, Michael. *Gide's Bent: Sexuality, Politics, Writing.* New York: Oxford University Press, 1995.

Luciano, Dana. *Arranging Grief: Sacred Time and the Body in Nineteenth-Century America.* New York: New York University Press, 2007.

MacIntyre, Alasdair. *After Virtue.* South Bend, Ind.: Notre Dame University Press, 1984.

Mains, Geoff. *Urban Aboriginals: A Celebration of Leathersexuality: 20th Anniversary Edition.* Los Angeles: Daedalus Publishing, 2002.

Martinac, Paula. *The Queerest Places: A National Guide to Gay and Lesbian Historic Sites.* New York: Henry Holt, 1997.

McGrath, Brian, with Mark Watkins and Mao-jung Lee. "There Is No *Queer Space,* Only Different Points of View." In *Queer Space* exhibition flyer. New York: Store Front for Art and Architecture, 1994. Unpaginated.

McNamara, Andrew. "Illegible Echoes: Felix Gonzalez-Torres, the Artist-Spy." *Image [&] Narrative* 22 (2008). http://www.imageandnarrative.be/inarchive/autofiction2/macnamara.htm.

Meat: True Homosexual Experiences from "Straight to Hell." San Francisco: Gay Sunshine Press, 1981.

Mendelsohn, Daniel. *The Elusive Embrace: Desire and the Riddle of Identity.* New York: Knopf, 1999.

Meyer, Richard. *Outlaw Representation: Censorship and Homosexuality in Twentieth-Century American Art.* New York: Oxford University Press, 2002.

Miller, Neil. *In Search of Gay America: Women and Men in a Time of Change.* New York: Atlantic Monthly Press, 1989.

———. *Out in the World: Gay and Lesbian Life from Buenos Aires to Bangkok.* New York: Random House, 1992.

Mitchell, Danielle. "Producing Containment: The Rhetorical Construction of Difference in *Will & Grace.*" *Journal of Popular Culture* 38 (2005): 105–6.

———. "Rhetorically Contained: The Construction and Incorporation of Difference in *Will & Grace.*" In *Rhetorical Agendas: Political, Ethical, Spiritual,* ed. P. Bizzell, 275–80. Mahwah, N.J.: Erlbaum, 2006.

Mohr, Richard D. "Architects of Identity." *The Guide* (May 1998). http://www.guidemag.com/magcontent/invokemagcontent.cfm.

Moore, Patrick. *Beyond Shame: Reclaiming the Abandoned History of Radical Gay Sexuality.* Boston: Beacon Press, 2004.

Mordden, Ethan. *How Long Has This Been Going On?* New York: Villard Books, 1995.

Mulvey, Laura. *Visual and Other Pleasures.* Bloomington: Indiana University Press, 1989.

Muñoz, José Esteban. *Cruising Utopia: The Then and There of Queer Futurity.* New York: New York University Press, 2009.

———. "Thinking beyond Antirelationality and Antiutopianism in Queer Critique." *PMLA* 21, no. 3 (May 2006): 825–26.

Munt, Sally. "The Lesbian Flâneur." In Bell and Valentine, *Mapping Desire,* 114–25.

Nahas, Rebecca, and Myra Turley. *The New Couple: Women and Gay Men.* New York: Seaview, 1979.

Nealon, Christopher. *Foundlings: Lesbian and Gay Historical Emotion Before Stonewall.* Durham, N.C.: Duke University Press, 2001.

Newton, Esther. *Cherry Grove, Fire Island: Sixty Years in America's First Gay and Lesbian Town.* New York: Basic, 1993.

———. "Role Models." 1972. In *Camp Grounds: Style and Homosexuality,* ed. David Bergman, 39–53. Amherst: University of Massachusetts Press, 1993.

Nickas, Robert. "Felix Gonzalez-Torres: All the Time in the World." *Flash Art* 24, no. 161 (Nov./Dec. 1991): 86–89.

Nora, Pierre. "Between Memory and History: Les Lieux de mémoire." Trans. Marc Roudebush. *Representations* 26 (Spring 1989): 7–24.

———, ed. *Les Lieux de mémoire,* 7 vols. Paris: Edition Gallimard, 1984–1992.

Nyong'o, Tavia. *The Amalgamation Waltz: Race, Performance, and the Ruses of Memory.* Minneapolis: University of Minnesota Press, 2009.

Pater, Walter. *Studies in the Renaissance.* 1873. London: Macmillan, 1914.

Patton, Cindy. *Inventing AIDS.* New York: Routledge, 1990.

Peake, Linda. "Race and Sexuality: Challenging the Patriarchal Structure of Urban Social Space." *Environment and Planning D* 11 (1993): 420–32.

Rechy, John. *The Sexual Outlaw: A Documentary.* New York: Grove, 1977.

Reed, Christopher. *Art and Homosexuality: A History of Ideas.* New York: Oxford University Press, 2011.

———. "Imminent Domain: Queer Space in the Built Environment." *Art Journal* 55, no. 4 (Winter 1996): 64–70.

———. "Pleasure Manifesto" *Queer Caucus for Art Newsletter* 15, no. 1 (January 2003) [archived at http://artcataloging.net/glc/qcano31].

———. "A Third Chicago School?" In *Chicago Architecture: Histories, Revisions, Alternatives,* ed. Katerina Rae Reudi and Charles Waldheim, 163–75. Chicago: University of Chicago Press, 2005.

Ricco, John. "Coming Together" *A/R/C* 1, no. 5 (Winter 1994–5): 26–31.

———. "The Itinerancy of Erotic Uncertainty." Paper delivered at the Society of Architectural Historians conference, Los Angeles, April 18, 1998, and at the University of Chicago, May 26, 1998.

Riley, Terence. *The Un-Private House.* New York: Museum of Modern Art, 1999.

Rist, Darrell Yates. *Heartlands: A Gay Man's Odyssey across America.* New York: Dutton, 1992.

Robbins, Mark. *Angles of Incidence.* New York: Princeton Architectural Press, 1992.

———. *Households.* New York: Monacelli Press, 2006.

Rochlitz, Rainer. *The Disenchantment of Art: The Philosophy of Walter Benjamin.* Trans. Jane Marie Todd. New York: Guildford Press, 1996.

Rodriguez, Suzanne. *Wild Heart, A Life: Natalie Clifford Barney's Journey from Victorian America to the Literary Salons of Paris.* New York: HarperCollins, 2002.

Román, David. "Remembering AIDS: A Reconsideration of the Film *Longtime Companion.*" *GLQ* 12, no. 2 (2006): 282–302.

Roof, Judith. "Generational Difficulties; or, The Fear of a Barren History." In *Generations: Academic Feminists in Dialogue,* ed. Devoney Looser and E. Ann Kaplan, 69–87. Minneapolis: University of Minnesota Press, 1997.

Roscoe, Will, ed. *Radically Gay: Gay Liberation in the Words of Its Founder, Harry Hay.* Boston: Beacon Press, 1996.

Rosenfeld, Israel. *The Invention of Memory: A New View of the Brain.* New York: Basic, 1988.

Ross, Andrew. *No Respect: Intellectuals and Popular Culture.* New York: Routledge, 1989.

Rubin, Gayle. "The Leather Menace: Comments on Politics and S/M." 1981. In Escoffier, *Sexual Revolution,* 266–99.

Rushdie, Salman. *The Wizard of Oz.* London: British Film Institute, 1992.

Ruskin, Cindy. *The Quilt: Stories from the NAMES Project.* New York: Pocket, 1988.

Russo, Vito. *The Celluloid Closet: Homosexuality in the Movies.* New York: Harper & Row, 1981.

———. "Why We Fight." Speech delivered at ACT UP Demonstrations in Albany, New York, May 9, 1988, and at the Department of Health and Human Services, Washington, D.C., October 10, 1988. http://www.actupny.org.

Saint, Andrew. "Philip Johnson: Flamboyant Postmodern Architect Whose Career Was Marred by a Flirtation with Nazism." *Guardian* (London), January 29, 2005, 25.

Sanders, Joel, ed. *Stud: Architectures of Masculinity.* New York: Princeton Architectural Press, 1996.

Saslow, James. *Pictures and Passions: A History of Homosexuality in the Visual Arts.* New York: Viking, 1999.

———. "A Sculpture without a Country." *Christopher Street* 5, no. 4 (February 1981): 23–32.

Savage, Todd. "The Metropolis Observed." *Metropolis Magazine* (July 1999). http://www.metropolismag.com/html/content_0799.

Schiappa, Edward. *Beyond Representational Correctness: Rethinking Criticism of Popular Media.* Albany: State University of New York Press, 2008.

Schulze, Franz. "Chicago Now." *Art in America* (September 1998): 63.

Schwartz, Frederick, ed. *Alan Buchsbaum, Architect and Designer: The Mechanics of Taste.* New York: Monacelli Press, 1996.

Scott, A. O. "'Chuck and Buck': Childhood Longings in a Grown-Up World." *New York Times,* July 14, 2000. http://www.nytimes.com/library/film/071400chuck-film-review.html.

Sedgwick, Eve Kosofsky. *Between Men: English Literature and Male Homosocial Desire.* New York: Columbia University Press, 1985.

———. *Epistemology of the Closet.* Berkeley: University of California Press, 1990.

———. "Paranoid Reading and Reparative Reading; or, You're So Paranoid, You Probably Think This Introduction Is about You." In *Novel Gazing: Queer Readings in Fiction,* ed. Eve Kosofsky Sedgwick, 1–37. Durham, N.C.: Duke University Press, 1997.

Sember, Robert. "In the Shadow of the Object: Sexual Memory in the AIDS Epidemic." *Space and Culture* 6, no. 3 (August 2003): 214–34.

"Sex Clubs and Bathhouses again Popular with Some Gay Men." National Public Radio, *All Things Considered,* June 1, 1995.

Shively, Charley. "Indiscriminate Promiscuity as an Act of Revolution." 1974. In *Gay Roots: Twenty Years of Gay Sunshine,* ed. Winston Leyland, 257–63. San Francisco: Gay Sunshine Press, 1991.

———. "Introduction." In *Meat: True Homosexual Experiences from "Straight to Hell,"* 5–8.

Smallwood, Lola. "Gay-Pride Halsted Street Project Ends in Harmony." *Chicago Tribune* November 15, 1998, sec. 4, 3.

Snediker, Michael. *Queer Optimism: Lyric Personhood and Other Felicitous Persuasions.* Minneapolis: University of Minnesota Press, 2009.

Sontag, Susan. "Notes on Camp." 1964. In *Against Interpretation and Other Essays,* 277–94. New York: Dell, 1969.

Spector, Nancy. *Felix Gonzalez-Torres.* New York: Simon Guggenheim Museum, 1995.

Stockton, Kathryn Bond. *The Queer Child, or Growing Sideways in the Twentieth Century.* Durham, N.C.: Duke University Press, 2009.

Stein, Marc. *City of Sisterly and Brotherly Loves: Lesbian and Gay Philadelphia, 1945–1972.* Chicago: University of Chicago Press, 2000.

Stolberg, Sheryl Gay. "Gay Culture Weighs Sense and Sexuality." *New York Times,* November 23, 1997.

Strong, Lester. "Coloring the World Queer." *Delmas Howe: Stations, A Gay Passion.* New York: Leslie/Lohman Gay Art Foundation, 2007. Unpaginated.

Sturken, Marita. "Narratives of Recovery: Repressed Memory as Cultural Memory." In Bal, Crewe, and Spitzer, *Acts of Memory,* 231–48.

———. *Tangled Memories: The Vietnam War, the AIDS Epidemic, and the Politics of Remembering.* Berkeley: University of California Press, 1997.

Summers, Claude. "George Segal's *Gay Liberation.*" *glbtq: an encyclopedia of gay, lesbian, bixesual, transgender, & queer culture.* http://www.glbtq.com/arts/george_1s.

"Surprise, Surprise." *Chicago Free Press,* November 29, 2000, 2.

Symonds, John Addington. *Studies of the Greek Poets.* 2 vols. London: Smith, Elder and Co., 1873.

"Theorizing Queer Temporalities: A Roundtable Discussion." *GLQ* 13, no. 2–3 (2007): 177–95.

Third World Gay Revolution (Chicago) and Gay Liberation Front (Chicago). "Gay Revolution and Sex Roles." In *Out of the Closets: Voices in Gay Liberation,* ed. Karla Jay and Allen Young, 252–58. New York: New York University Press, 1992.

Thompson, E. P. "Time, Work-Discipline, and Industrial Capitalism." *Past & Present* 38, no. 1 (1967): 56–97.

Tucker, Ernest. "'Gay Pride' Street Markers Get a Toning Down." *Chicago Sun Times,* November 1, 1997, 1.

Urbach, Henry. "Spatial Rubbing: The Zone." *Sites* 25 (1993): 90–95.

Usborne, David. "Gay LA." *Architectural Design* 43 (August 1973): 567.

Vaid, Urvashi. "Last Word: Panic or Panacea?" *The Advocate* 748 (December 9, 1997): 88.

Valentine, Gill. "Out and About: Geographies of Lesbian Landscapes." *International Journal of Urban Regional Research* 19, no. 1 (1995): 96–111.

Vidal, Gore. *Point to Point Navigation: A Memoir 1964–2006.* New York: Doubleday, 2006.

Video Remains. Dir. Alexandra Juhasz. 2005.

Vogtherr, Christoph Martin. "Absent Love in Pleasure Houses: Frederick II of Prussia as Art Collector and Patron." In *Other Objects of Desire: Collectors and Collecting Queerly,* ed. Michael Camille and Adrian Rifkin, 69–82. Oxford: Blackwell, 2001.

von Agoston, Alexander. "Belmont." *Off the Rocks* 12 (2005): 78–79.

Von Franz, Marie-Louise. *Puer Aeternus.* Boston: Sigo Press, 1981.

Walters, Suzanna Danuta. *All the Rage: The Story of Gay Visibility in America.* Chicago: University of Chicago Press, 2001.

Warner, Michael. "Media Gays: A New Stone Wall." *The Nation,* July 14, 1997, 15–19.

———. *The Trouble with Normal: Sex, Politics, and the Ethics of Queer Life.* New York: Free Press, 1999.

Wäspe, Roland. "Private and Public." In *Felix Gonzalez-Torres,*" 1:18–21.

Watney, Simon. *Imagine Hope: AIDS and Gay Identity.* London: Routledge, 2000.

———. "Short-Term Companions: AIDS as Popular Entertainment." In *A Leap in the Dark: AIDS, Art & Contemporary Cultures,* ed. Allan Klusacek and Ken Morrison, 152–66. Montreal: Vehicule Press, 1992.

Weightman, Barbara A. "Gay Bars as Private Places." *Landscape* 23 (1980): 9–16.

Weiner, Lori. "North Halsted Project Stirs Up Support, and Controversy, among Gay and Non-Gay Residents, Business Owners." *Outlines* (September 1997). http://www.windycitymediagroup.com/archives/current/outlines/archives/090397/halsted.

Weisman, Leslie Kanes. *Discrimination by Design: A Feminist Critique of the Man-Made Environment.* Urbana: University of Illinois Press, 1992.

Weston, Kath. "Get Thee to a Big City: Sexual Imaginary and the Great Gay Migration." *GLQ* 2 (1995): 253–77.

Whitney, Catherine. *Uncommon Lives: Gay Men and Straight Women.* New York: Plume, 1990.

Wilde, Oscar. *Intentions.* 1891. New York: Brentano's, 1912.

Wolfe, Maxine. "Invisible Women in Invisible Places: Lesbians, Lesbian Bars, and the Social Production of People/Environment Relationships." *Architecture and Behavior* 8, no. 2 (1992): 137–58.

Young, James E. "The Counter-Monument: Memory Against Itself in Germany Today." 1992. In *Art and the Public Sphere,* ed. W. J. T. Mitchell, 49–78. Chicago: University of Chicago Press, 1992.

Younge, Gary. "White History 101." *Nation* 5 (March 2007). http://www.thenation.com/article/white-history-101.

INDEX

CHRISTOPHER CASTIGLIA is Liberal Arts Research Professor of English at the Pennsylvania State University. He is the author of *Bound and Determined: Captivity, Culture-Crossing, and White Womanhood from Mary Rowlandson to Patty Hearst* and *Interior States: Institutional Consciousness and the Inner Life of Democracy* and coeditor with Glenn Hendler of Walt Whitman's temperance novel, *Franklin Evans; or, The Inebriate.*

CHRISTOPHER REED is professor of English and visual culture at the Pennsylvania State University. He is the author of *Bloomsbury Rooms: Modernism, Subculture, and Domesticity* and *Art and Homosexuality: A History of Ideas;* the editor of *Not at Home: The Suppression of Domesticity in Modern Art and Architecture* and *A Roger Fry Reader;* editor and translator of *The Chrysanthemum Papers: "The Pink Notebook of Madame Chrysanthemum" and Other Documents of French Japonisme;* and coeditor with Nancy Green of the exhibition catalog *A Room of Their Own: The Bloomsbury Artists in American Collections.*